THE
MAYO CLINIC

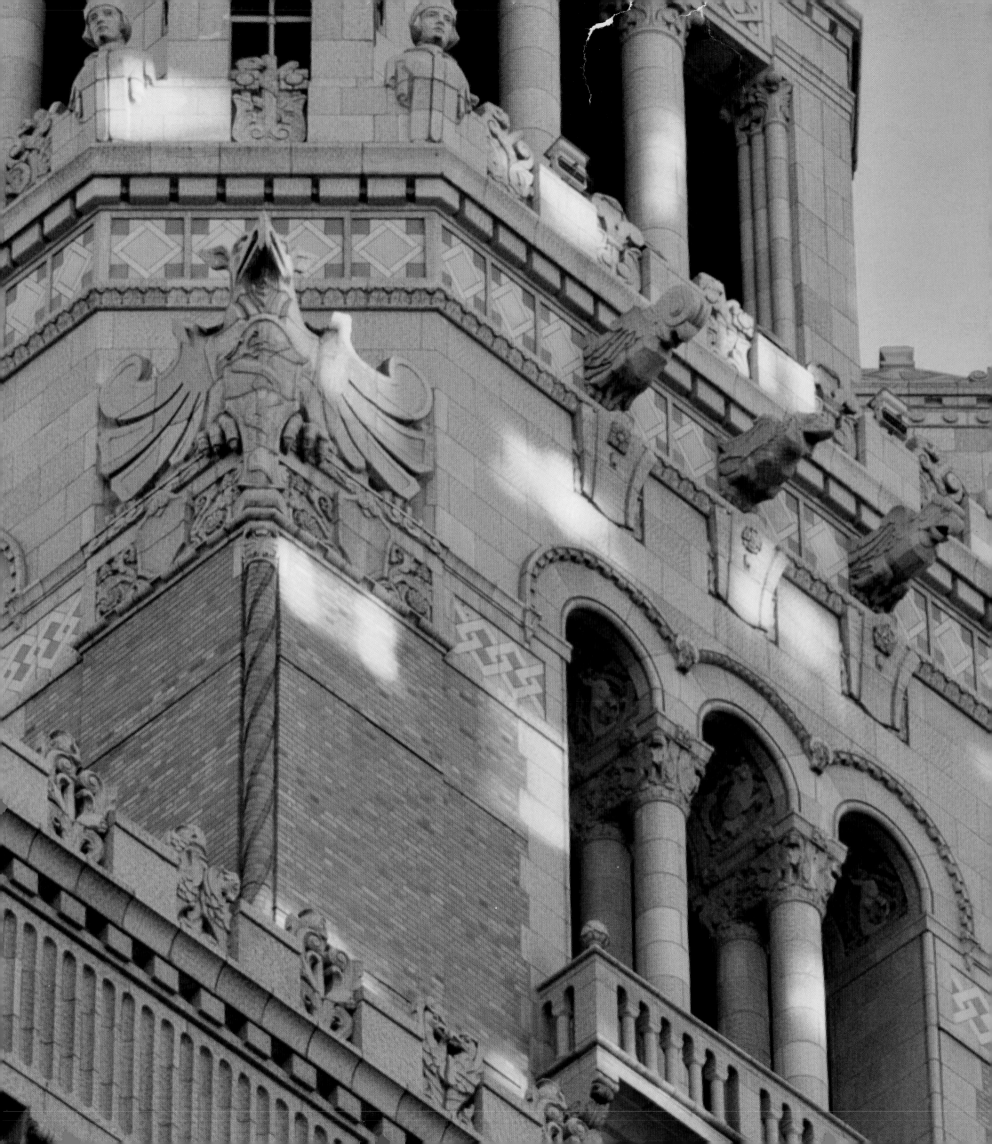

THE
MAYO CLINIC

FAITH · HOPE · SCIENCE

PUBLISHED BY

RosettaBooks®

CEO: Arthur Klebanoff

ISBN-13: 9781948122290
Library of Congress Control Number: 2018947058

First Edition 2018
Printed in the United States of America
10 9 8 7 6 5 4 3 2 1

Ewers Brothers Productions, LLC/Florentine Films
Written by: David Blistein, Ken Burns
Creative Consultants: Ken Burns, Erik Ewers,
    Christopher Loren Ewers, Julie Coffman, David Blistein
Project Liaison: Rebecca Connolly
Cover Art: Brian Lee
Legal Services: Drew Patrick

**Oxmoor House, an imprint of Time Inc. Books,
a division of Meredith Corporation**
Editor: Sarah Rutledge
Assistant Editor: April Colburn
Senior Manager, Business Development
    and Partnerships: Nina Reed
Project Editor: Lacie Pinyan
Designer: Jon Chaiet
Assistant Production and Project Manager: Kelsey Smith
Indexer: Jay Kreider

Mayo Clinic
Senior Product Manager: Christopher Frye
Director, Heritage Hall: Matthew Dacy
Communications Manager: Robert Nellis
Chair, Public Affairs: Chris Gade
Coordinator, Public Affairs: Beth Backus
Editorial Research Librarians: Erika Riggin, Abbie Brown
Administrative Assistants: Jennifer Conrad, Paula Graskamp,
    Terri Zanto Strausbach

The sum total of medical knowledge is now so great and wide spreading that it would be futile for...any one man to assume that he has even a good working knowledge of any large part of the whole. The very necessities of the case are driving practitioners into cooperation. The best interest of the patient is the only interest to be considered, and in order that the sick may have the benefit of advancing knowledge, union of forces is necessary.

—DR. WILL MAYO

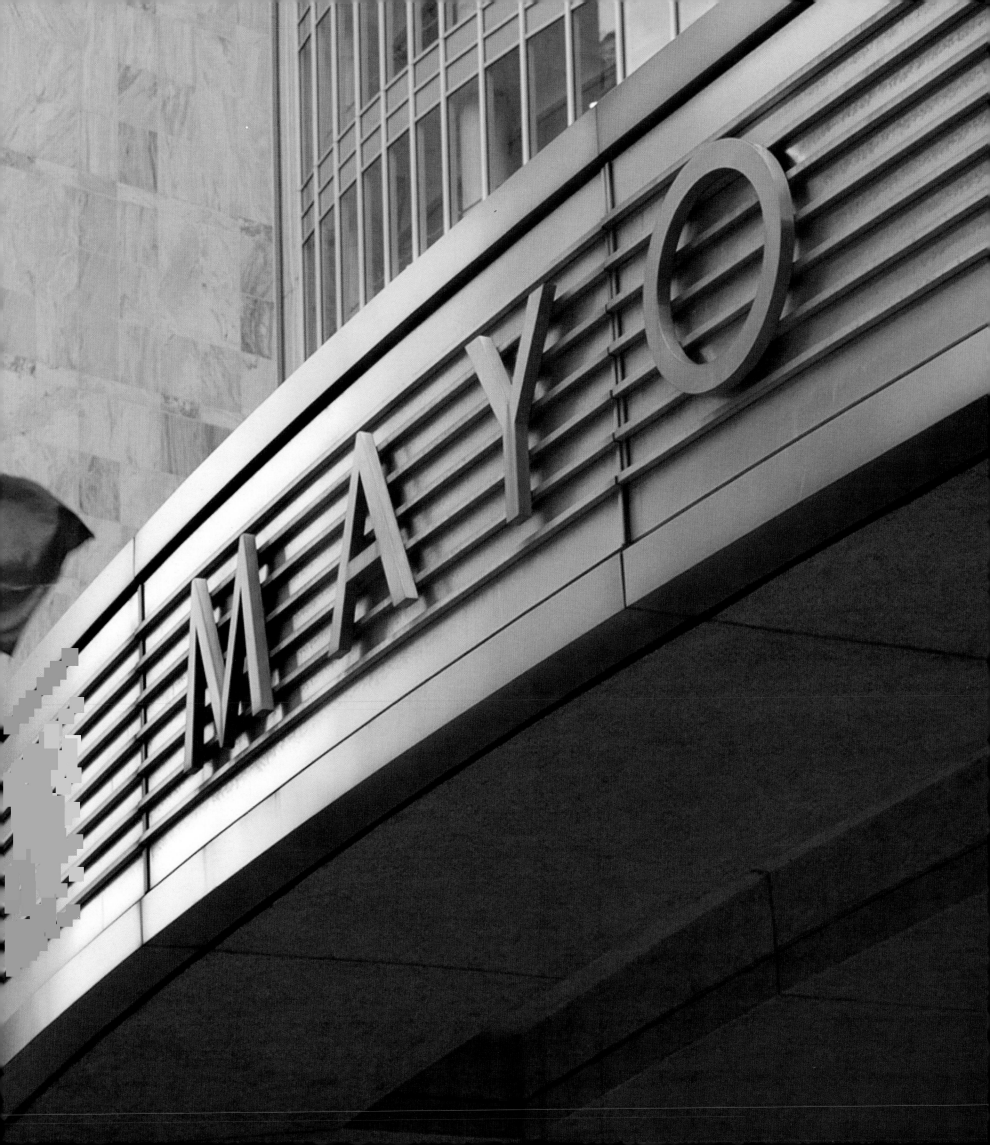

TEAMWORK IN HEALTH CARE AND FILMMAKING

I have admired the films of Ken Burns all my adult life.

When the topic arose of a film about Mayo Clinic, Ken made it clear that he and his team required absolute editorial freedom. Mayo would have no oversight or control. From the Mayo Clinic perspective, we completely agreed, knowing how informed outsiders would bring the objectivity and credibility that audiences deserve.

Ken brought his longtime collaborators, Ewers Brothers Productions, to this project: co-director and editor Erik Ewers, co-director and cinematographer Christopher Loren Ewers, producer Julie Coffman and writer David Blistein. It has been inspiring to witness how the filmmakers and the staff of Mayo Clinic share a dedication to service, creativity and technical excellence.

Throughout the project, Ken and his colleagues followed the story where it took them, across our campuses in Minnesota, Florida and Arizona. Mayo Clinic opened its doors and archives; our patients and staff opened their hearts. Ken and his team members were with us at the memorial service for Sister Generose Gervais, the last Franciscan Sister to serve as chief hospital administrator, and for a long list of innovative procedures, including early cancer treatments using proton beam therapy and breakthrough surgeries for pancreatic cancer.

Teamwork is the hallmark of Mayo Clinic. Every day, more than 60,000 colleagues unite their diverse skills to serve patients and advance medical science. It was a new experience for our staff to have another type of team embedded with us—one that focused on filmmaking.

When we asked what they'd like to see, the film team replied, "Everything." So, for nearly three years, we took them from our subways to the rooftops. They had help from our Center for the History of Medicine, the Sisters of Saint Francis, an advisory panel representing all sectors of Mayo Clinic, the Mayo family, the personnel of our historic homes and Mayo facilities staff—at all hours of the day and night. Our video team provided every bit of film footage we have of the Mayo brothers and assisted with equipment and logistics when needed. This crew spent more time in surgery than any non-Mayo film crew in history. We never said no to any request.

The resulting film, *The Mayo Clinic: Faith, Hope, Science*, along with this companion book, capture what Dr. Will Mayo called "the spirit of the Clinic." We are particularly grateful to the film's benefactors, whose generous support made the project possible.

On behalf of the patients we serve, and everyone who looks to Mayo Clinic for hope and healing, it is a privilege to share this story with you.

John H. Noseworthy

John H. Noseworthy, M.D.
President and Chief Executive Officer
Mayo Clinic

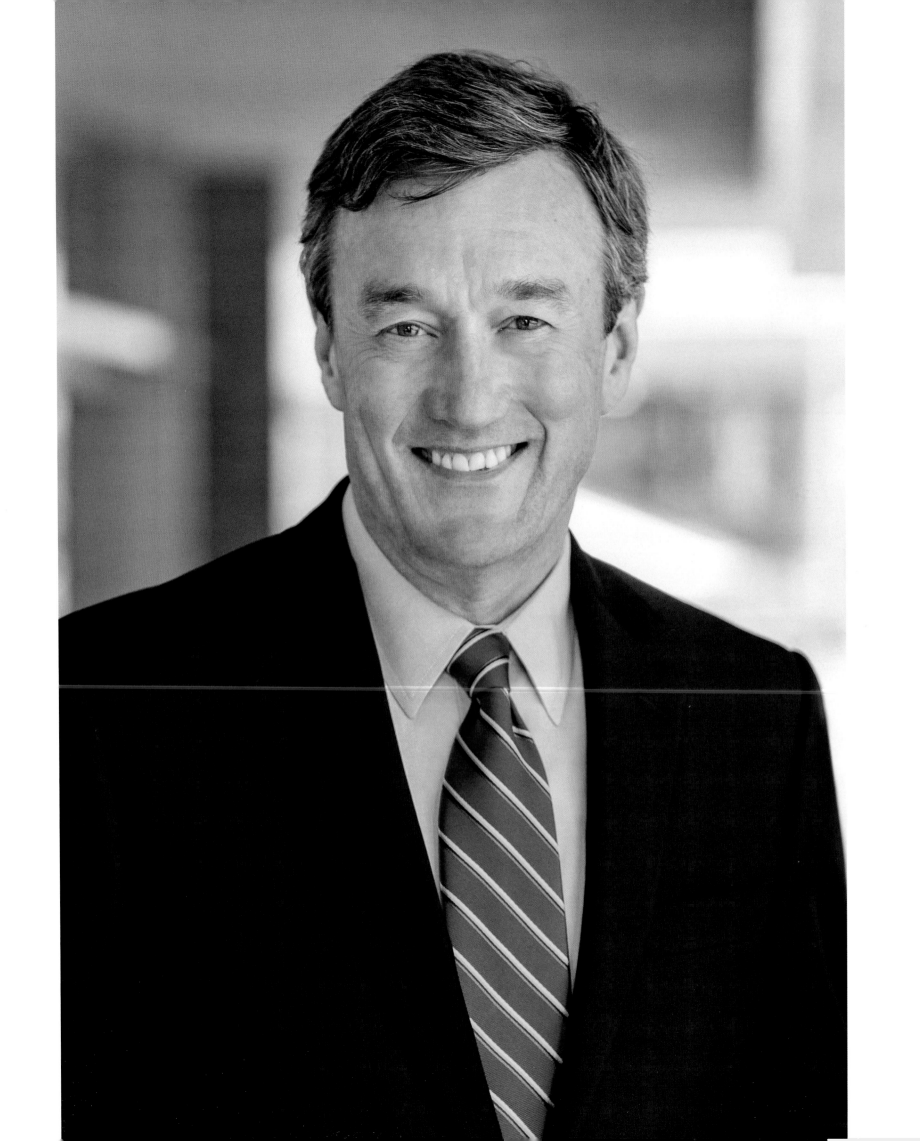

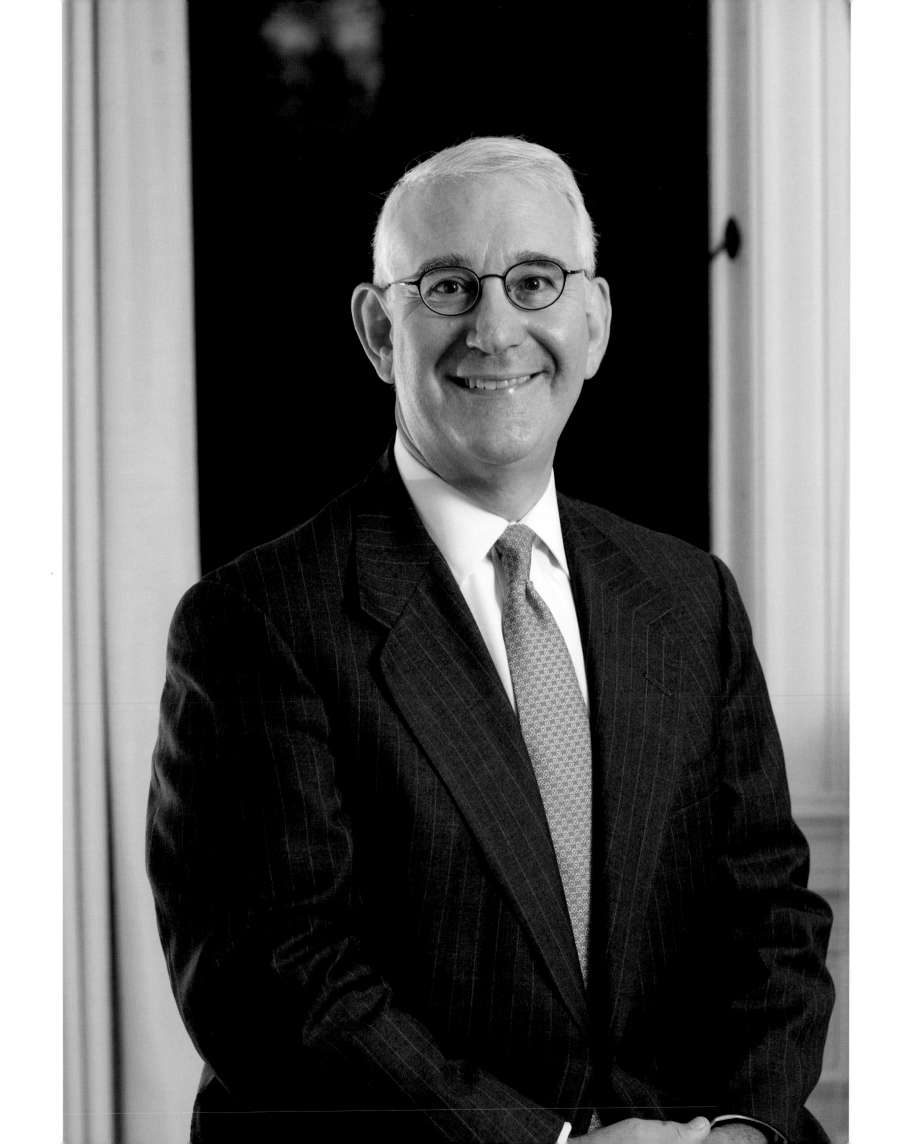

MAYO CLINIC IS AN AMERICAN ICON

As a patient and friend of Mayo Clinic, and in my service as chair of the Board of Trustees, I am delighted to welcome you to this companion volume of the film by Ken Burns and Ewers Brothers Productions, *The Mayo Clinic: Faith, Hope, Science.*

The Board of Trustees is the ultimate governing authority of Mayo Clinic, which officially approved Mayo's cooperation in the project. Members represent a wide range of professional backgrounds in fields such as academia, business, government and the news media.

We share the conviction that Mayo Clinic is an American icon. Mayo represents the highest ideals of the United States, yet is open to the world. Mayo is unique, yet offers a philosophy and best practices worthy of emulation. Mayo Clinic's primary value, "The needs of the patient come first," has guided the organization's remarkable contributions to health care throughout its history and will be equally important in the years ahead.

People turn to Mayo Clinic for care of complex conditions and hard-to-diagnose diseases. In 2017, Mayo served 1.3 million patients from all 50 states and 136 countries. Millions more benefit as Mayo makes discoveries, communicates information and educates the next generation of skilled, compassionate health-care professionals.

And it all began with a family of country doctors and an order of Catholic Sisters who were schoolteachers. A natural disaster in 1883 made them unlikely partners in healing. The frontier spirit of mutual support and innovation led them to create an entirely new way of practicing medicine.

This is a story that needs to be told.

My colleagues on the Board were delighted when Ken Burns and his associates, consummate filmmakers of integrity and unparalleled quality, stepped forward. The film was made possible by generous production underwriter support. It has been a pleasure to see their work unfold over the course of several years.

As the film says, "For 150 years, the Mayo Clinic has been confronting age-old questions about our commitment to taking care of each other, about the role of money and profit in medicine, and about the very nature of healing itself." The timing of this production is significant, because despite all the changes that have taken place in Mayo's history, seismic shifts are yet to come. Rapidly advancing medical knowledge and technical capabilities are juxtaposed with issues of access, affordability and privacy. The role of the individual—patient as well as caregiver—must be determined in the context of the larger society that includes family, community and government. Ethics and values have profound impact in an arena whose essence is human life.

Mayo Clinic has an important voice in this conversation. When transforming their private practice into a not-for-profit organization dedicated to patient care, research and education, Dr. Will and Hattie Mayo, along with Dr. Charlie and Edith Mayo, signed a Deed of Gift. It said the "ultimate purposes" of Mayo Clinic, "past, present and future, must be measured largely by its contributions to the general good of humanity."

Throughout succeeding generations, the people of Mayo Clinic have endeavored to fulfill this public trust. I commend the Ken Burns and Ewers Brothers team for capturing the journey so eloquently through humane storytelling of the highest standard.

Samuel A. Di Piazza, Jr.
Chair, Mayo Clinic Board of Trustees

FOREWORD BY KEN BURNS

In late January 2015, I sat down with John Noseworthy and explained, in no uncertain terms, why he did not want me to do a film on Mayo Clinic. He had brought up the idea before, but—even though I had been a Mayo patient for years and I knew what an extraordinary place it was—I had always demurred. Still, I agreed to discuss it one more time.

First, I reminded him that my films are about people, not institutions. He nodded understandingly. Then I explained that I already had enough projects in the planning stages to keep me busy for the next fifteen years. Again, he nodded.

Then I told him the real reason the Mayo Clinic didn't want me to do the film: "You will have absolutely no creative say in the project."

"Understood," he said.

"We need total access to your locations, your people, your facilities."

"No problem," he said.

"We're not doing a film *for* the Mayo Clinic. We're doing a film *about* the Mayo Clinic. We tell stories. We don't take sides."

"Of course," he said.

"What if we discover something really bad?" I asked.

"If you discover it, we want to know about it."

I began to feel like W.W. Mayo after the tornado trying to explain to Mother Alfred why she shouldn't try to build a hospital! So we shook on it—sealing the deal the same way the Mayo brothers and Sisters of Saint Francis had for a century. The hospital was built. The film was made. And John was true to his word.

We were granted extraordinary access to people and places and archives. We experienced firsthand the spirit of cooperation and generosity that is at Mayo's core. And people spoke to us with unflinching honesty. More than once, a doctor, a nurse, a nun, or a patient broke down in tears during an interview.

I knew even back then that I had protesteth too much at the beginning. I make films about quintessentially American topics, and I can think of no story more quintessentially American than that of Mayo Clinic. At a time when we are trying to figure out how to fix an incredibly flawed health-care system, Mayo Clinic's history speaks to larger themes that transcend political arguments. Ultimately, it addresses the age-old question of what we owe each other in terms of how we care for one another. This quest was the original animating spirit of Mother Alfred, W.W. Mayo, and Mayo's sons. And it's still practiced there today.

Mayo does a lot of things right. Having doctors on salary is a good idea. It fosters collaboration and reduces unnecessary procedures. Having laboratory facilities alongside the surgical suites is a good idea. It greatly speeds up results and minimizes the need for additional operations. Putting the needs of the patient first is, of course, the best idea of all. It sounds so simple. And yet, at times, it's incredibly complex.

Mayo struggles with the same challenges as every other health-care organization today. Access is a real problem. One of the patients we followed had to wait almost a year to get an appointment. Insurance is another real problem. (The same patient worried about losing medical coverage when her husband lost his job.) Then there is the biggest challenge of all—the fact that every single day Mayo employees have to deal with matters of life and death. Early on, a surgeon really opened our eyes to the reality of health care when he told us that every physician has his or her own personal graveyard—people whose lives could not be saved. As we say in the film, "mistakes are made, people die."

Mayo is far more than a "clinic." It is far more than three campuses and a regional health-care system and a worldwide clinical-care network. It is far more even than the one million patients it sees every year and the thousands of employees who care for them. I like to say that our films explore the possibility that sometimes one and one equals three, that the whole can be so much more than the sum of its parts. I can't think of a better example than the relationship of the Sisters of Saint Francis and the Mayo brothers that this organization was built on. The faith of one plus the humility of the other. The dedication of one plus the commitment of the other. The intuition of one plus the intelligence of the other. Can you tell which is which? That's the point. The Sisters and the Mayo brothers each brought their own unique expression of those qualities to the table and, together, they created something bigger.

At the very beginning of this process, we had a simple question: What is Mayo Clinic? In fact, during one of our early screenings, I realized we were already one-third of the way through our story and we didn't even have a place we could call Mayo Clinic yet! There was just a doctors' practice led by two brothers named Mayo who did surgery at a hospital run by a small community of nuns.

So, for three years, we immersed ourselves in Mayo's history and everyday life. Co-director Erik Ewers interviewed everyone from grieving parents to the Dalai Lama; his co-director (and brother) Christopher Loren Ewers filmed enough operations to be a surgical assistant and enough sunrises to be a Minnesota farmer. Producer Julie Coffman got on a first-name basis with everyone from the doorman in Jacksonville to the CEO in Rochester. And writer David Blistein became an expert on everything from the Franciscan catechism to pharmacogenomics.

I've seen this film dozens and dozens of times and the images never fail to move me to my core. It's the same looking through this book. Lucy Gray, the little girl with the paper chain behind her bed; an impossibly huge proton-beam accelerator looming over tiny Abigail Feenstra; the brothers Mayo sitting in the back of an open car with President Franklin Delano Roosevelt; and concert violinist Roger Frisch, wide awake, his head in a harness on an operating table undergoing deep brain stimulation, drawing an absolutely steady bow across the strings for the first time in years.

People ask, "What's the secret sauce?" What unique combination of wisdom and values makes this organization so remarkable? We asked everyone we interviewed that very question.

Early in the film, a Mayo doctor comes as close as possible to giving out the recipe: "Medicine is a science," he told us. "But how we interact [with patients] is layered with all kinds of other issues—all of which have to do with health. And so, if they don't have faith in the caregivers, if that patient doesn't have hope, we're gonna have a lot of trouble, you know, even attempting to make them better. Faith, hope, and science, those things are absolutely critical."

As the Sisters would say, "Amen."

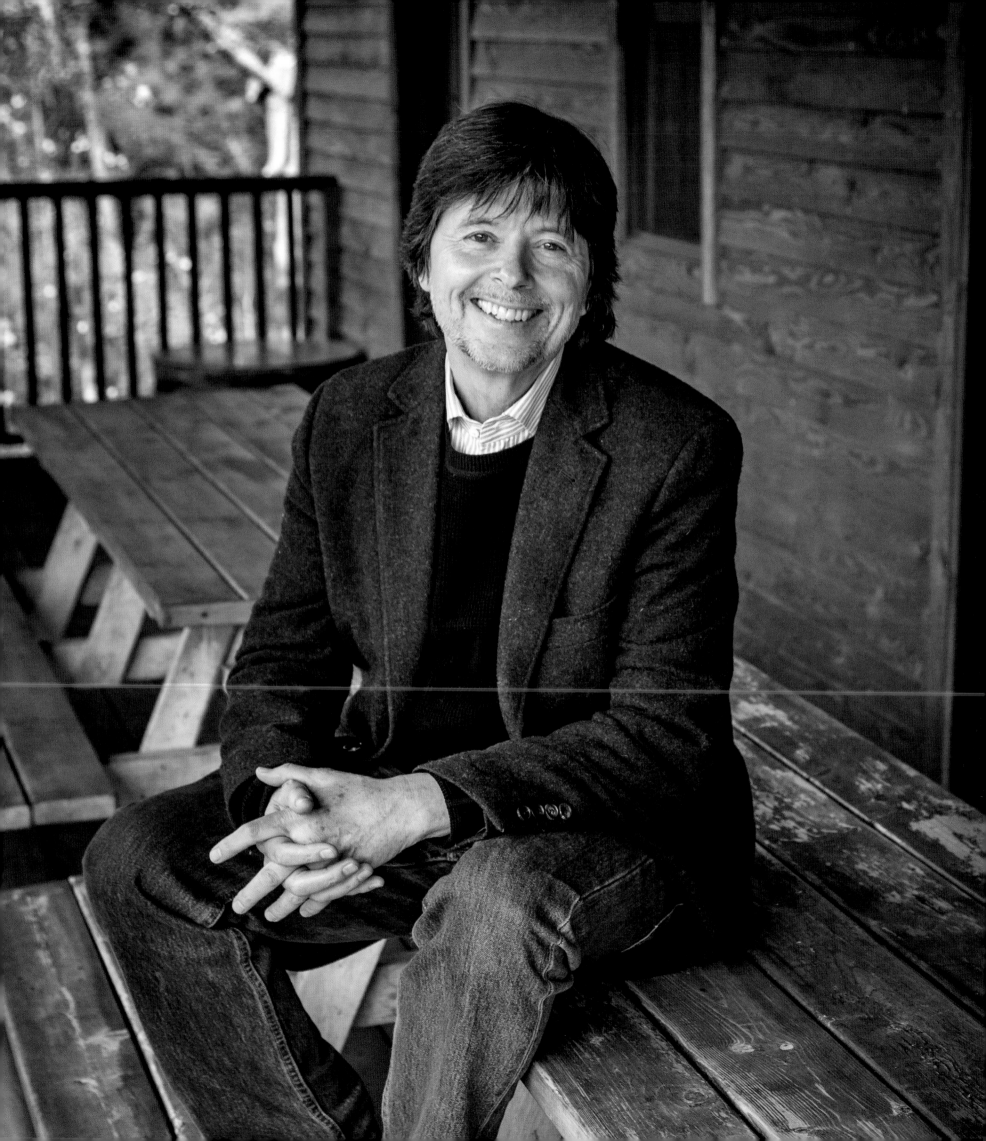

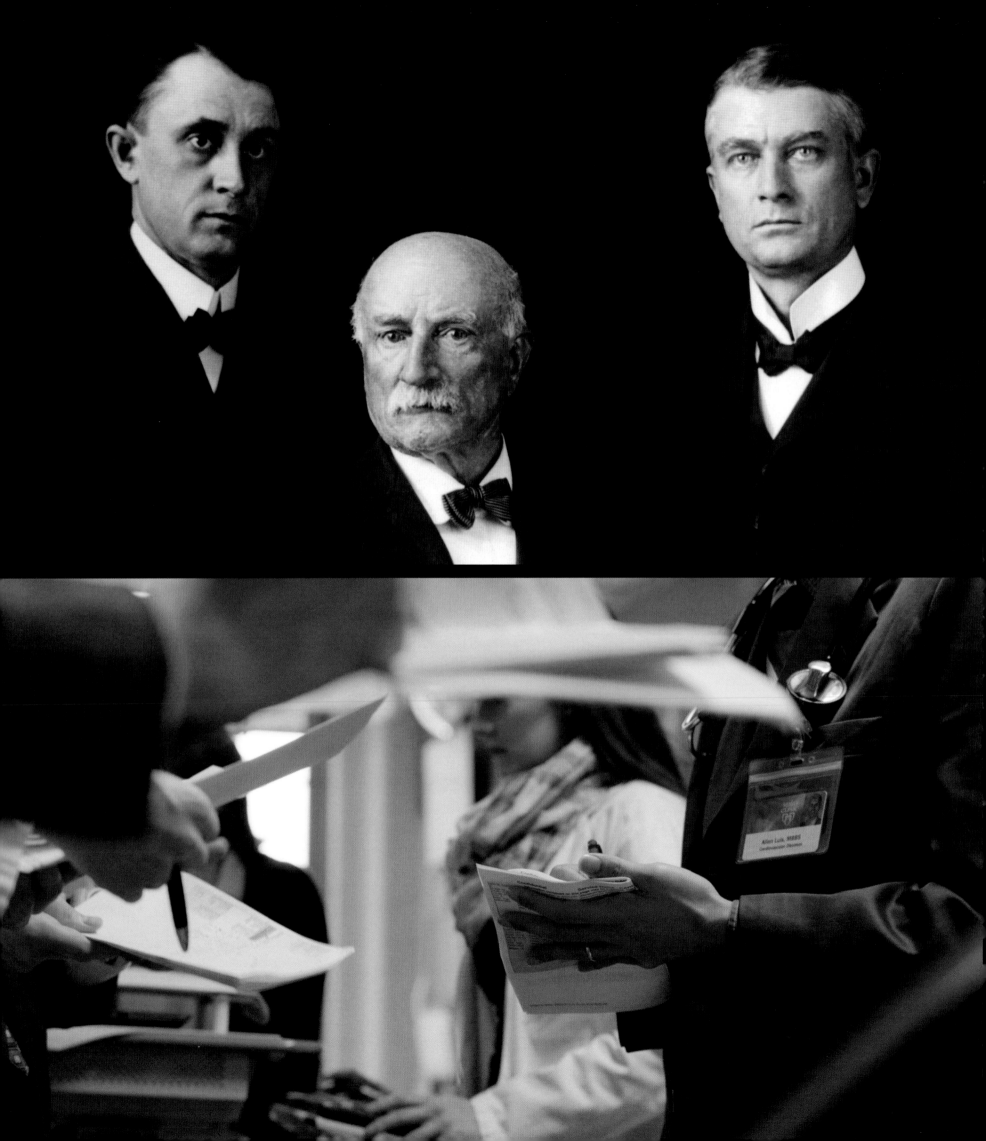

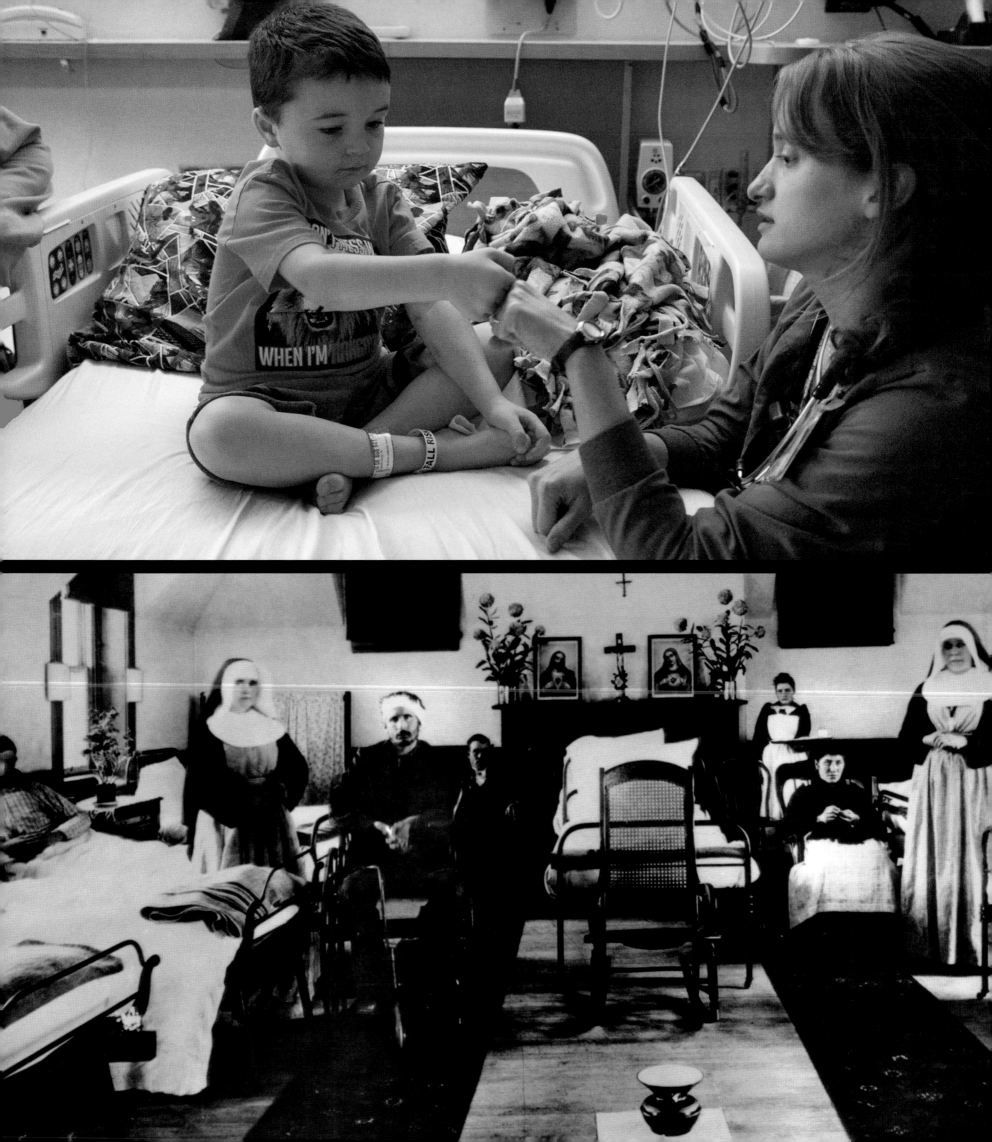

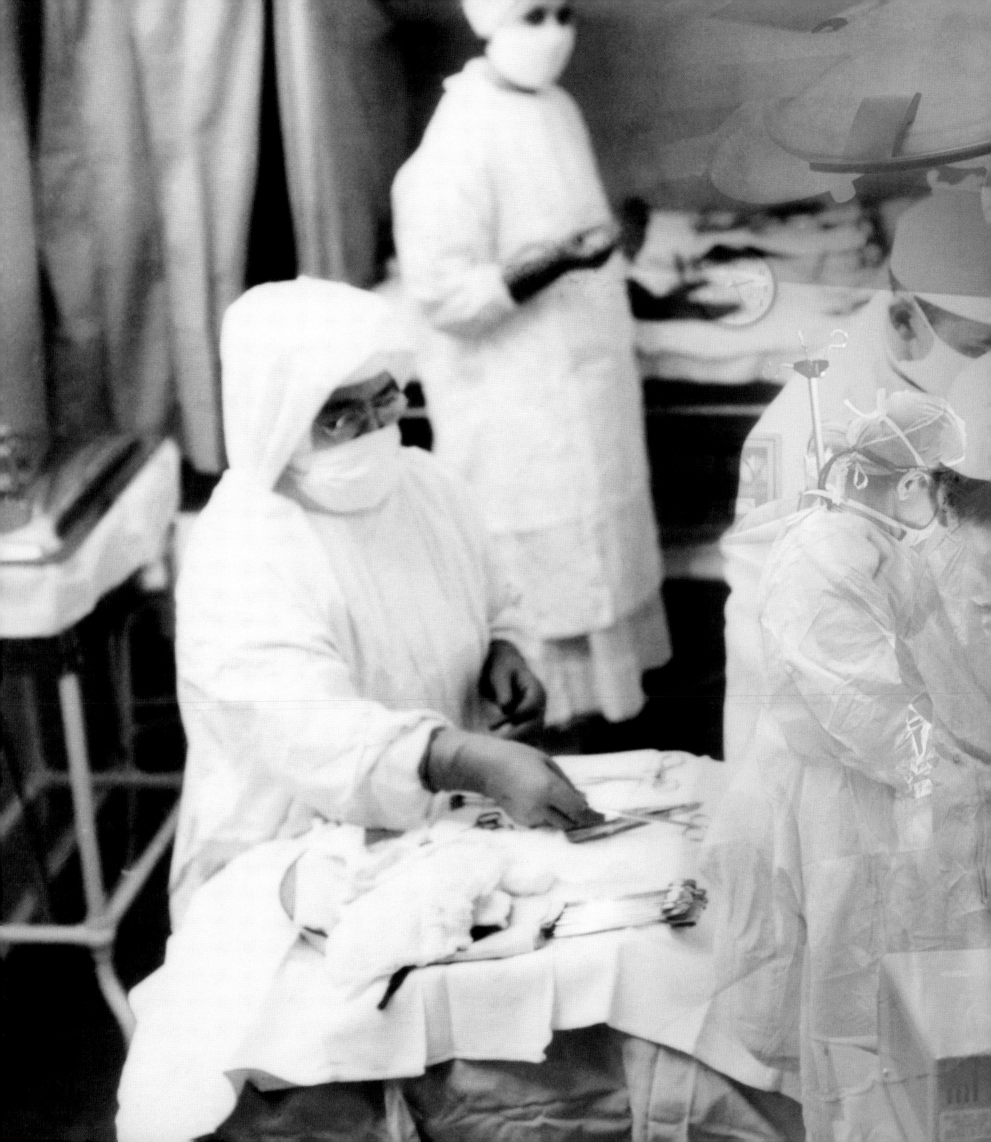

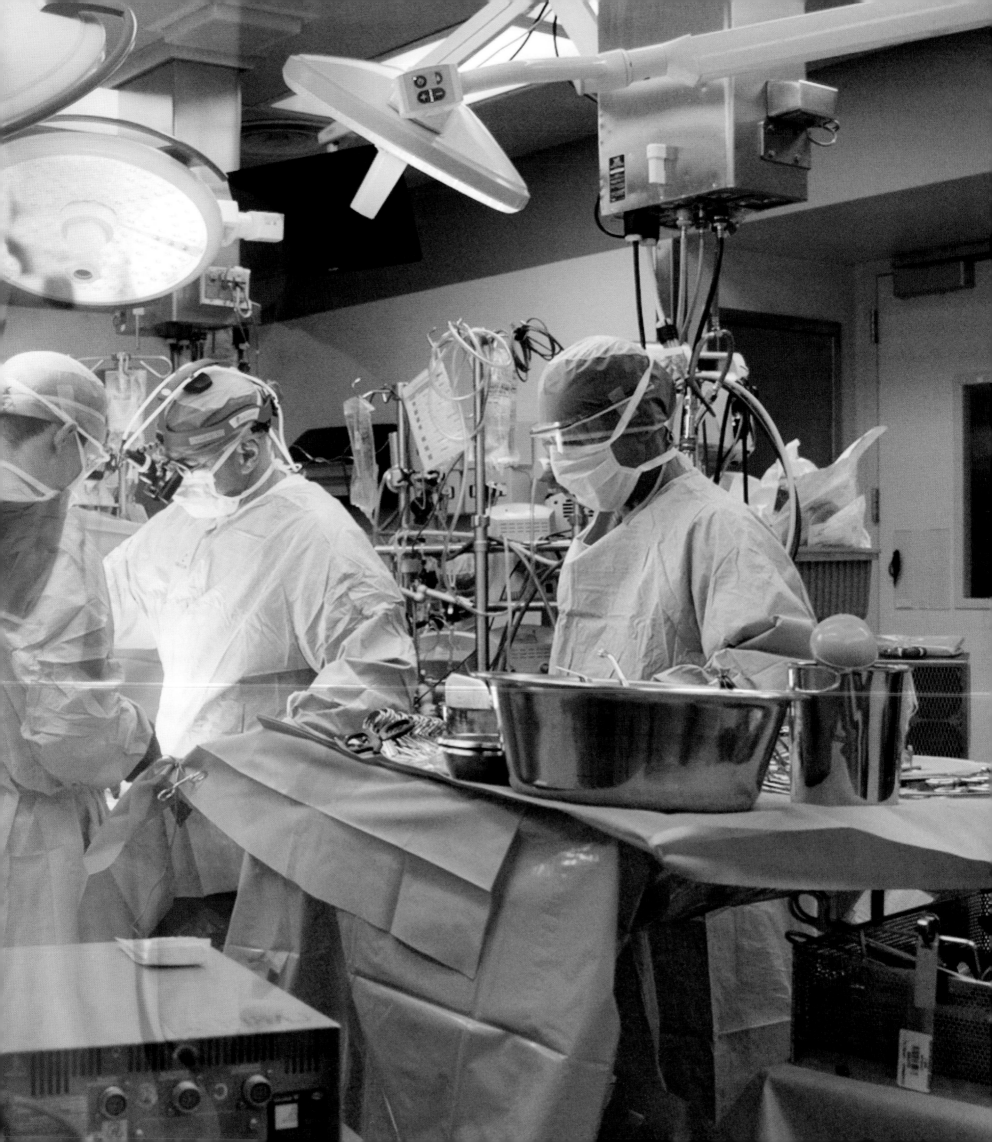

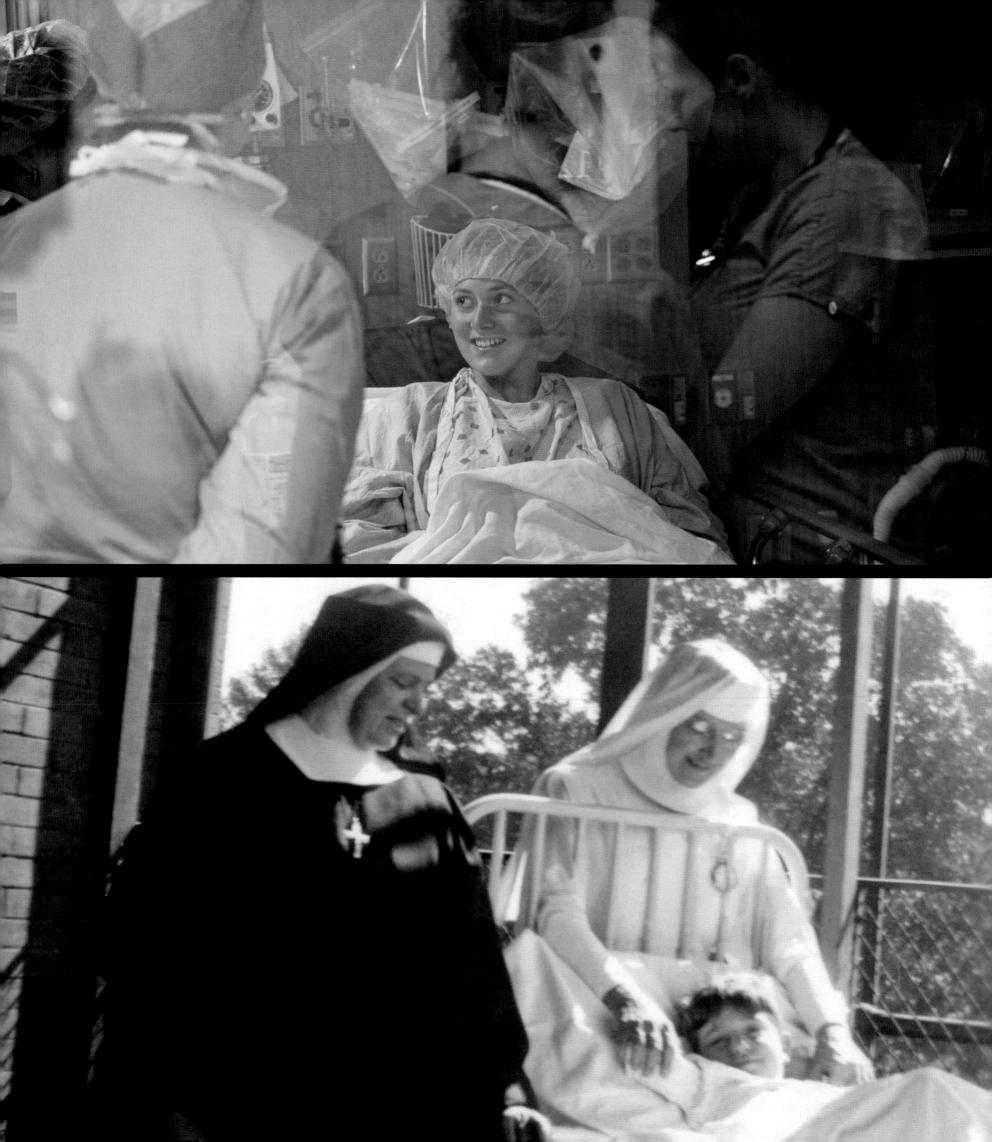

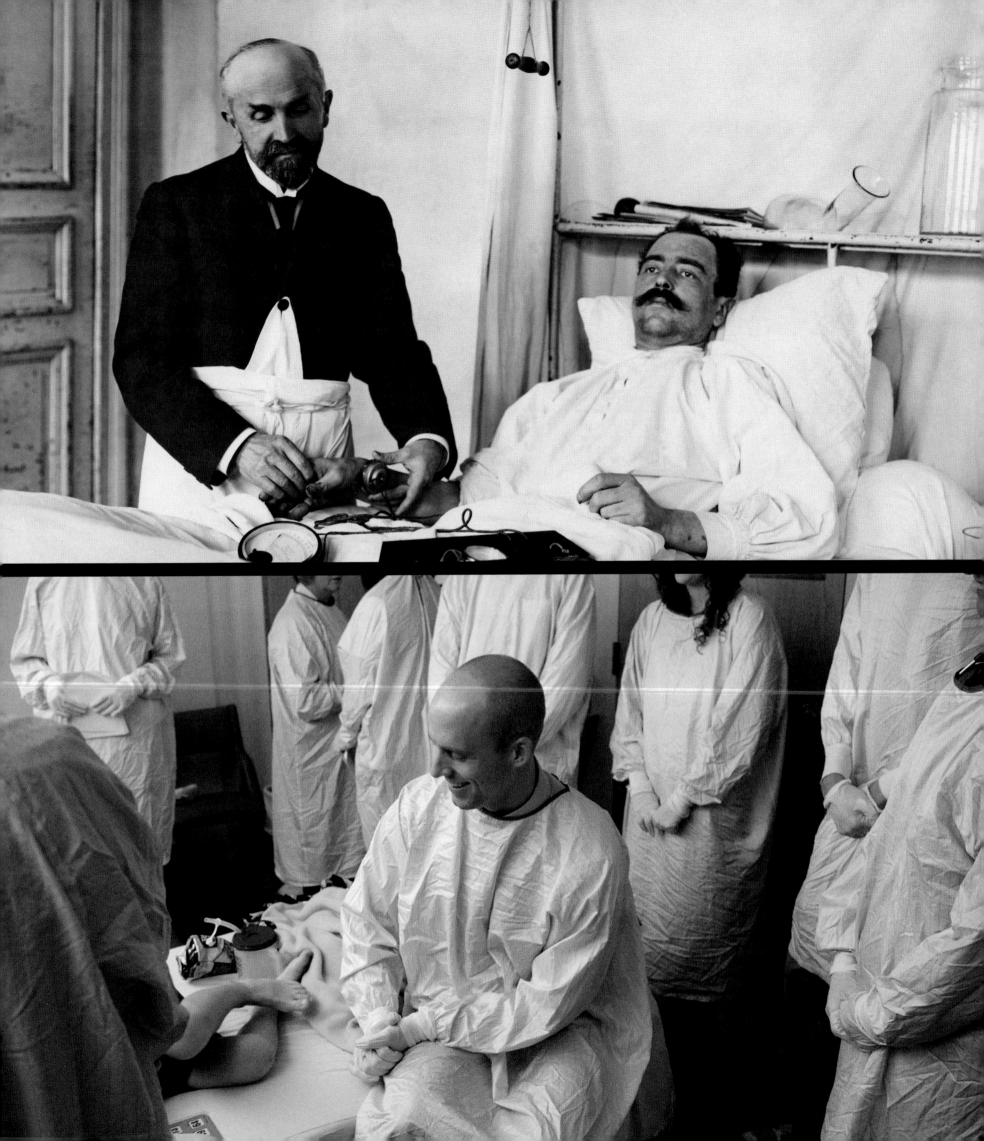

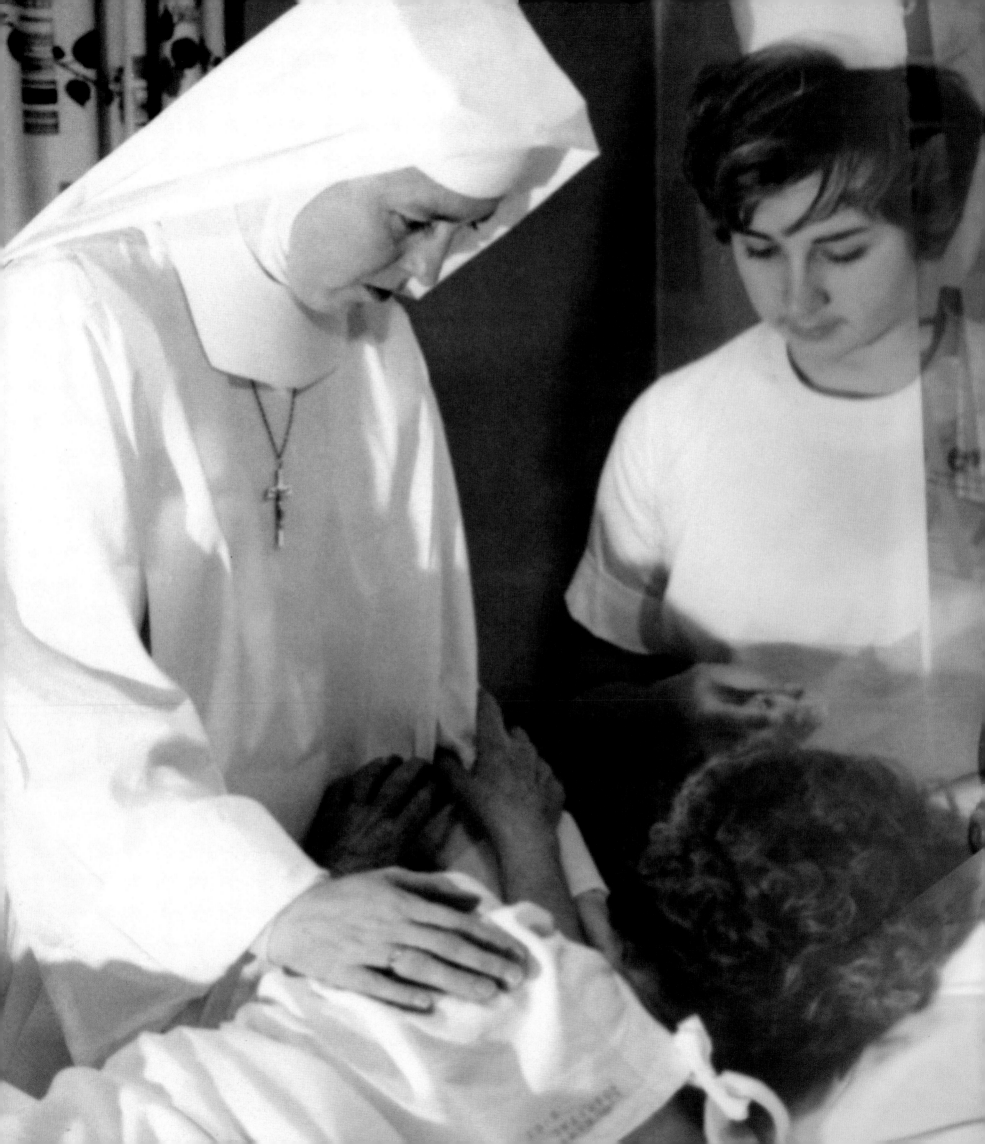

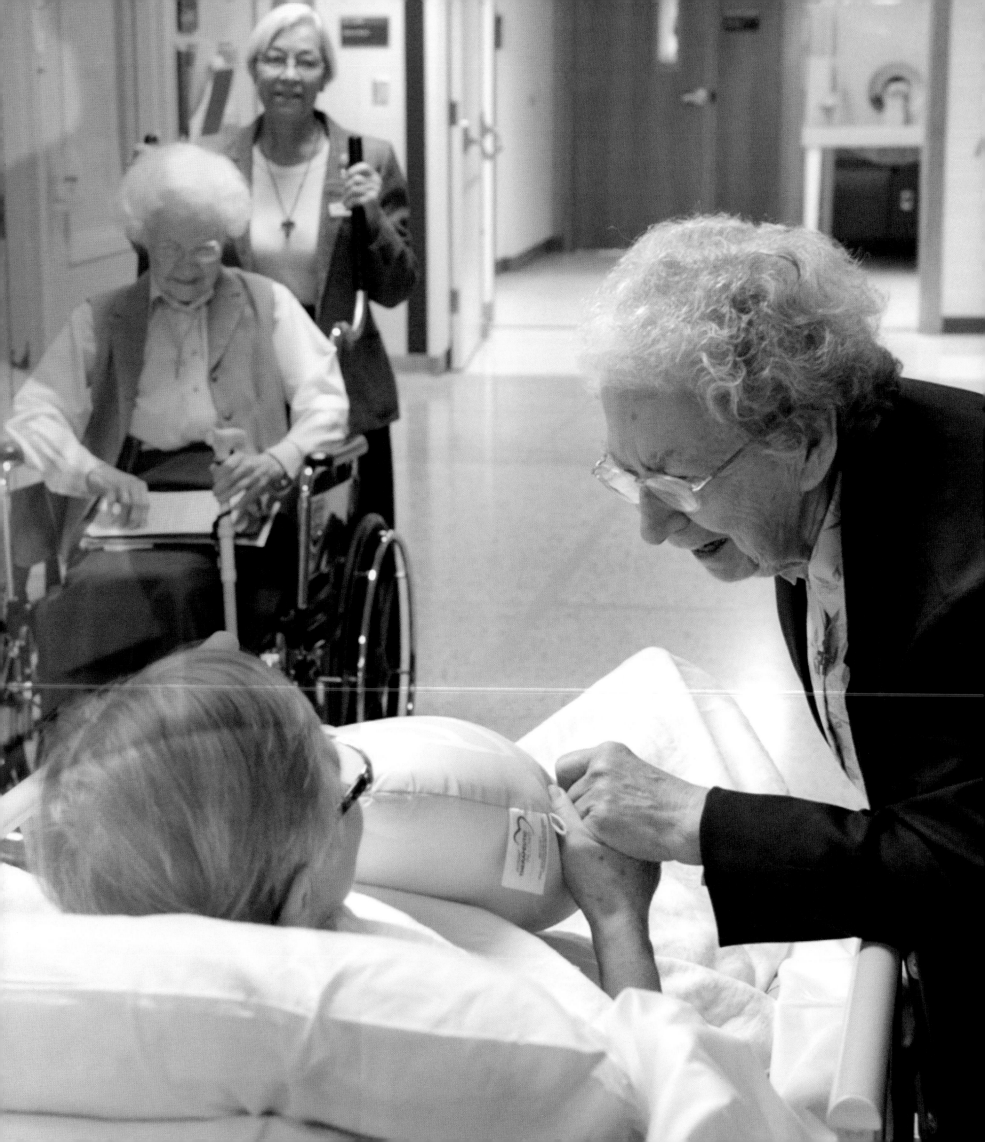

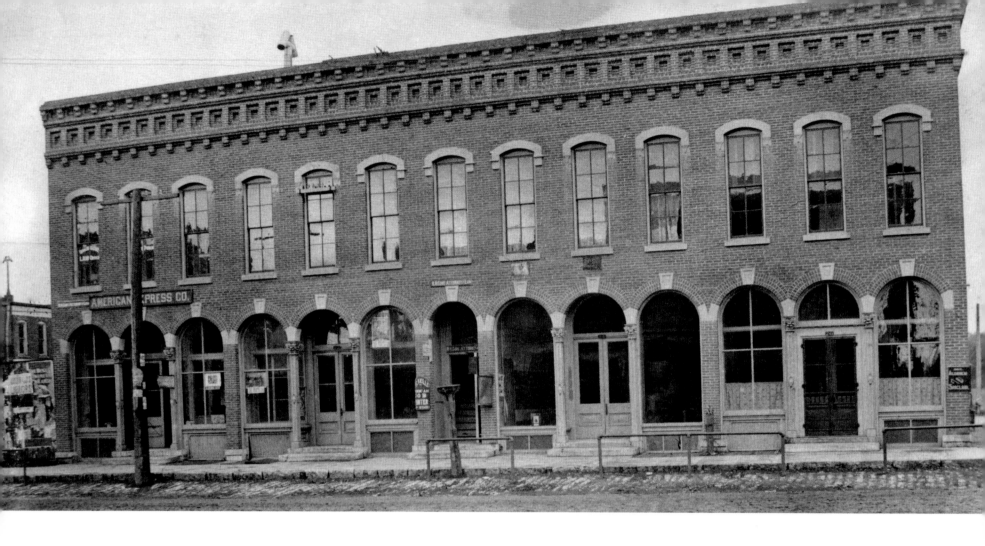

Imagine for a minute that you've been told that the doctors don't know what's wrong with you or can't help you. And then imagine if you will that you contact Mayo Clinic and Mayo Clinic says, "We can help you." Imagine what that does for that patient in terms of hope and inspiration and opportunity going forward for healing. That's what this place is about.

—JOHN NOSEWORTHY, M.D., PRESIDENT AND CEO, MAYO CLINIC

INTRODUCTION

On the early evening of August 21, 1883, Will and Charlie Mayo, the young sons of a local doctor in Rochester, Minnesota, were practicing eye surgery on a sheep's head at a slaughterhouse when the butchers urged them to go home immediately. A powerful storm was coming. One of the worst tornadoes in Minnesota history tore through the northern end of Rochester. Dr. William Worrall Mayo and his two sons treated scores of the wounded in homes, offices, hotels, even a dance hall. Amid the chaos, the elder Dr. Mayo asked to see Mother Alfred of the nearby Sisters of Saint Francis. It was summer—vacation time at the convent school she oversaw.

The students' rooms were empty, he said, could they use the beds for the injured? She agreed. Afterward, Mother Alfred told Dr. Mayo that she had received a vision from God instructing her to build a hospital in Rochester with Dr. Mayo as its director. It would become, she believed, "world renowned for its medical arts." Within a few years, Mother Alfred's vision—what people would call "the miracle in the cornfield"—came true. In one of the most unlikely partnerships, and in one of the most unlikely places, the Mayos and the Sisters of Saint Francis created what many believe is the greatest medical center in the world.

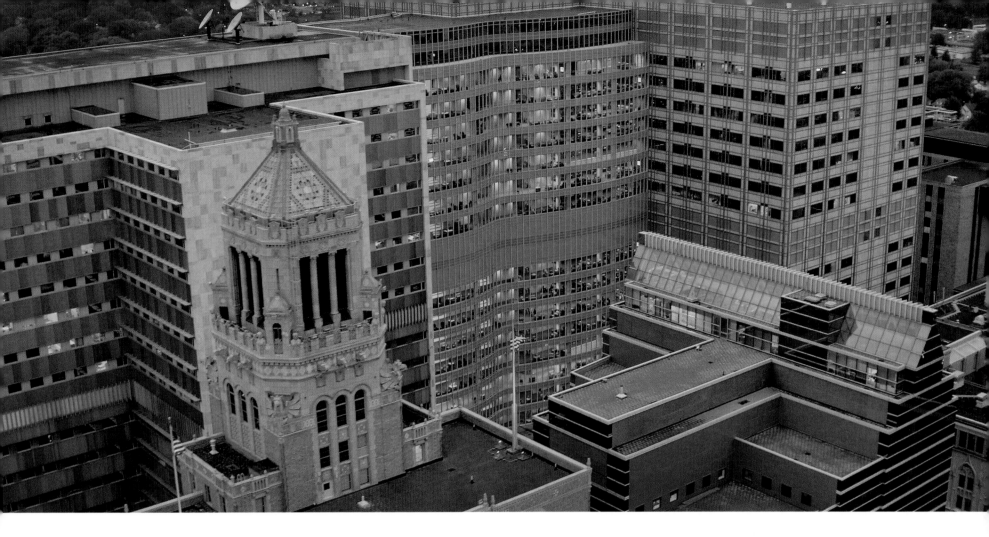

When William Worrall Mayo and his sons began practicing medicine together in Rochester, Minnesota, a small town ninety miles southeast of Minneapolis, there were only a handful of doctors in the whole county.

That three-person practice has grown into an organization employing more than 64,000 people, with campuses also in Florida and Arizona, and affiliates all over the world. For 150 years, Mayo Clinic has been confronting age-old questions about our commitment to taking care of each other, about the role of money and profit in medicine, and about the very nature of healing itself.

Each year more than a million patients arrive at Mayo Clinic from all 50 states and 150 countries. During any given 24-hour period as many as 14,000 patients will be seen; 9,000 examinations and 300 surgeries will be performed; 5,000 lab specimens will be evaluated; and 4,600 diagnostic procedures will be conducted, with 230 radiologists able to read the results and report back within 90 minutes. In an age when most doctors operate independently and are financially rewarded for ordering a battery of tests and procedures, every physician at Mayo Clinic is on salary, creating a culture that thrives on collaboration. Dr. Mayo had a simple philosophy he tried to impart to his sons: "The needs of the patient come first." They wouldn't treat diseases. They would treat people. And they would do it with the Sisters of Saint Francis.

I think that there is a reason so many people come to Mayo Clinic and have been for so many years. It has such a long history, and such a good reputation. Mayo was the right place to go and my parents could see that, too. When I first came, the history was powerful to me. We read the description of how it was built after the tornado. There was a sense of support in the history, and in the beliefs that those nuns had had that carries on today—not even in a religious sense; you just feel supported by that faith and hope.

—ANNA JENKINS,
PATIENT, DURHAM, NC

I was a child growing up in the Midwest, and the Mayo Clinic was a secular temple. It was something that we could all be proud of even if we had no association with it. And it was there in Rochester, Minnesota, like it had risen up out of the earth in some way.

—TOM BROKAW, PATIENT, ORIGINALLY FROM YANKTON, SD

Without losing hope, there's possibility to overcome. Our very life, you see, [is] based on hope, so hope is very, very important for our survival.

—DALAI LAMA, PATIENT, INDIA

Medicine is a science. But how we interact is layered with all kinds of other issues—all of which have to do with health. Faith, hope, and science, those things are absolutely critical.

—BRADLY NARR, M.D., MAYO CLINIC ANESTHESIOLOGIST

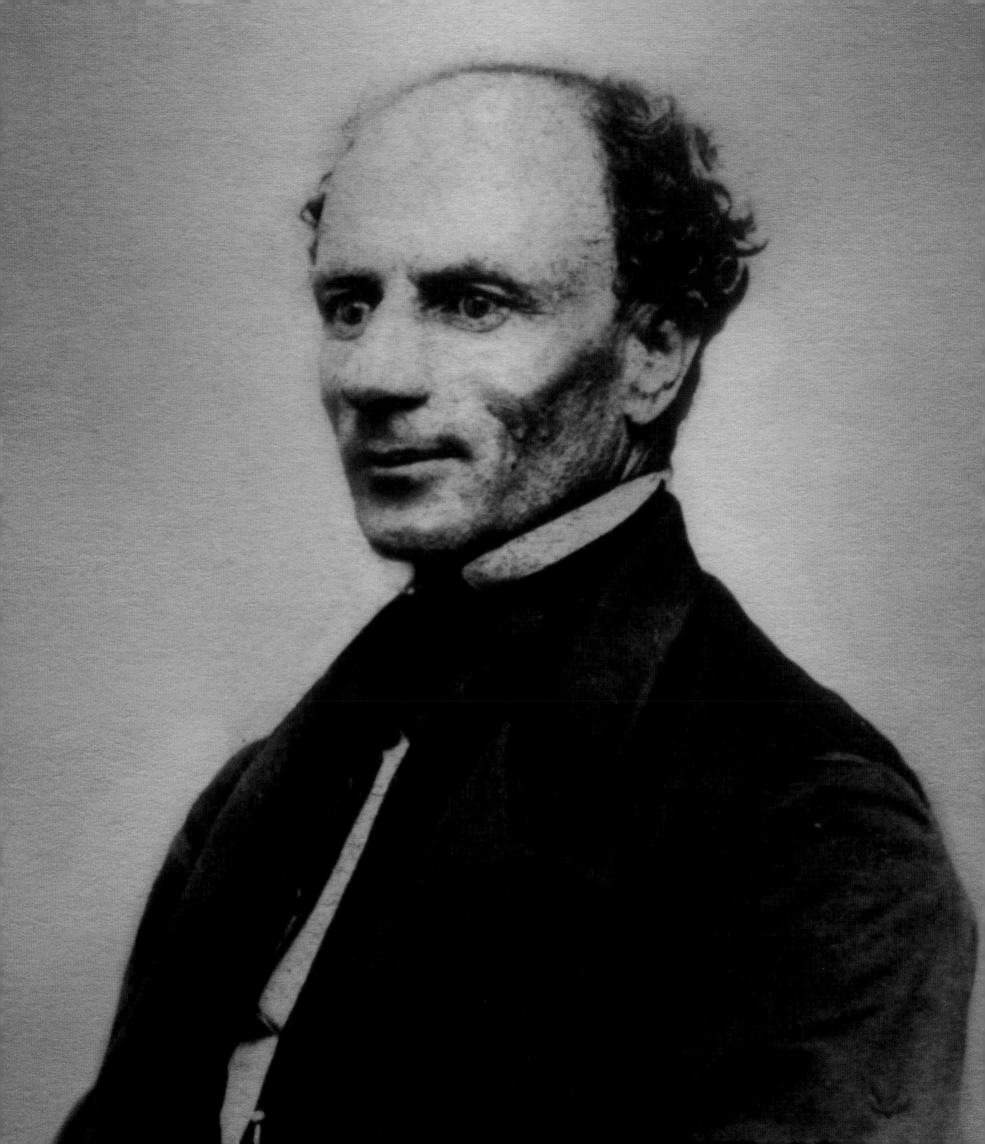

CHAPTER ONE

THE EDUCATION OF W.W. MAYO

My own religion has been to do all the good I could to my fellow man, and as little harm as possible.

—WILLIAM WORRALL MAYO, M.D.

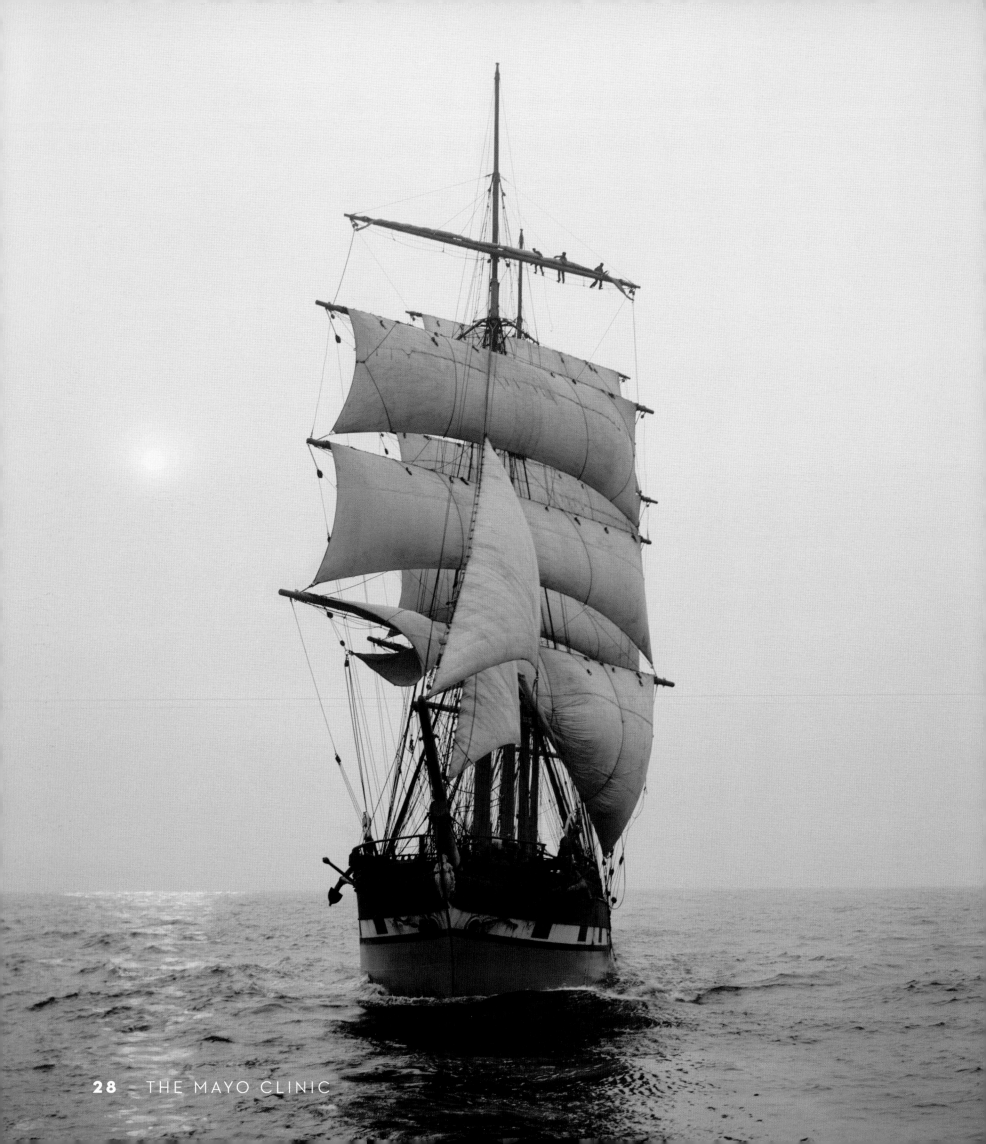

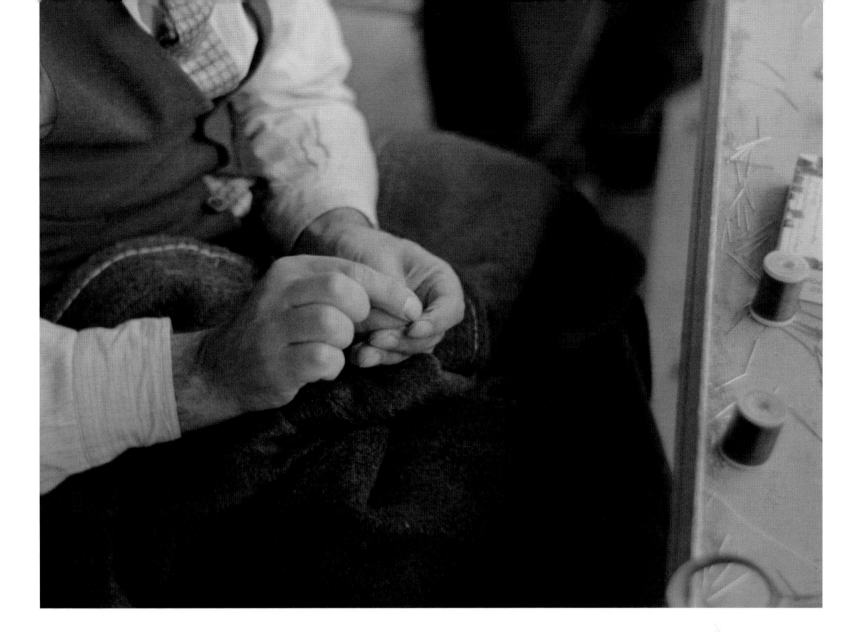

One day in 1846, a 27-year-old aspiring doctor named William Worrall Mayo went down to the docks in Liverpool, England, and got on a ship headed to America. He had been born in 1819 to a middle-class family near Manchester. His father was a cabinetmaker who died when his son was 7 years old, leaving his wife with six children to feed. At 14, W.W., as he would be known, became a tailor's apprentice, where he gained invaluable experience with a needle and thread.

W.W. Mayo was small (just 5'4"), wiry, and formal, with memorably piercing blue-gray eyes. One of his grandsons described him as "snap-tempered…strange, ferocious, striving, and restless." He studied with the famous chemist John Dalton, who promoted the theory that all matter is composed of atoms. Dalton was also a Quaker, and he instilled in W.W. a commitment to the scientific method, to hard work, and to social justice.

When W.W. arrived in America, his first job was as a chemist at Bellevue Hospital in New York City, where he saw the full range of human suffering.

[Hospitals] were places where the perception was, that's where you go to die. There really were almost no rules or regulations. They weren't sterile places. And there really weren't doctors as we perceive of them today. There were no standards, in terms of education, for individuals who claimed they were doctors. There were also a lot of quacks who toured the country proclaiming cures for this disease or that disease.

—BRUCE FYE, M.D., MAYO CLINIC
MEDICAL HISTORIAN

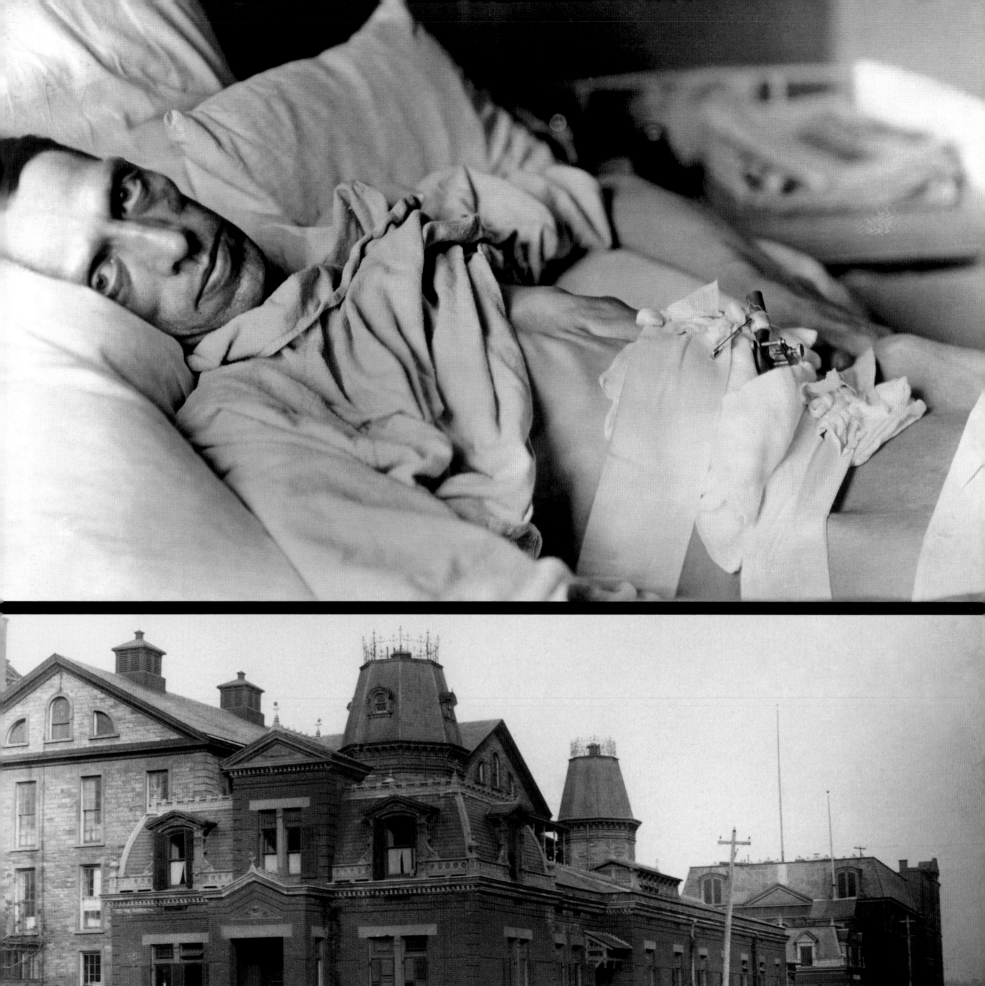

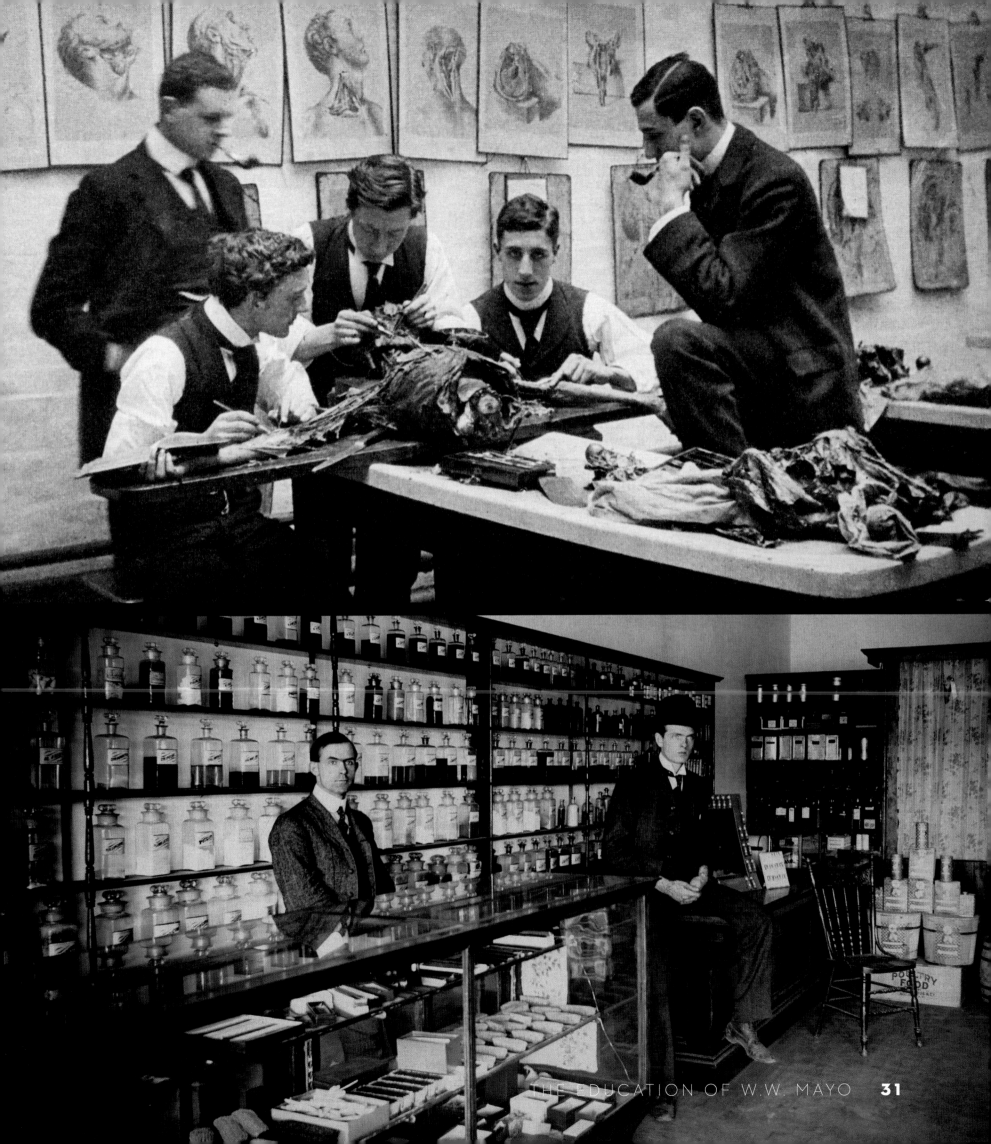

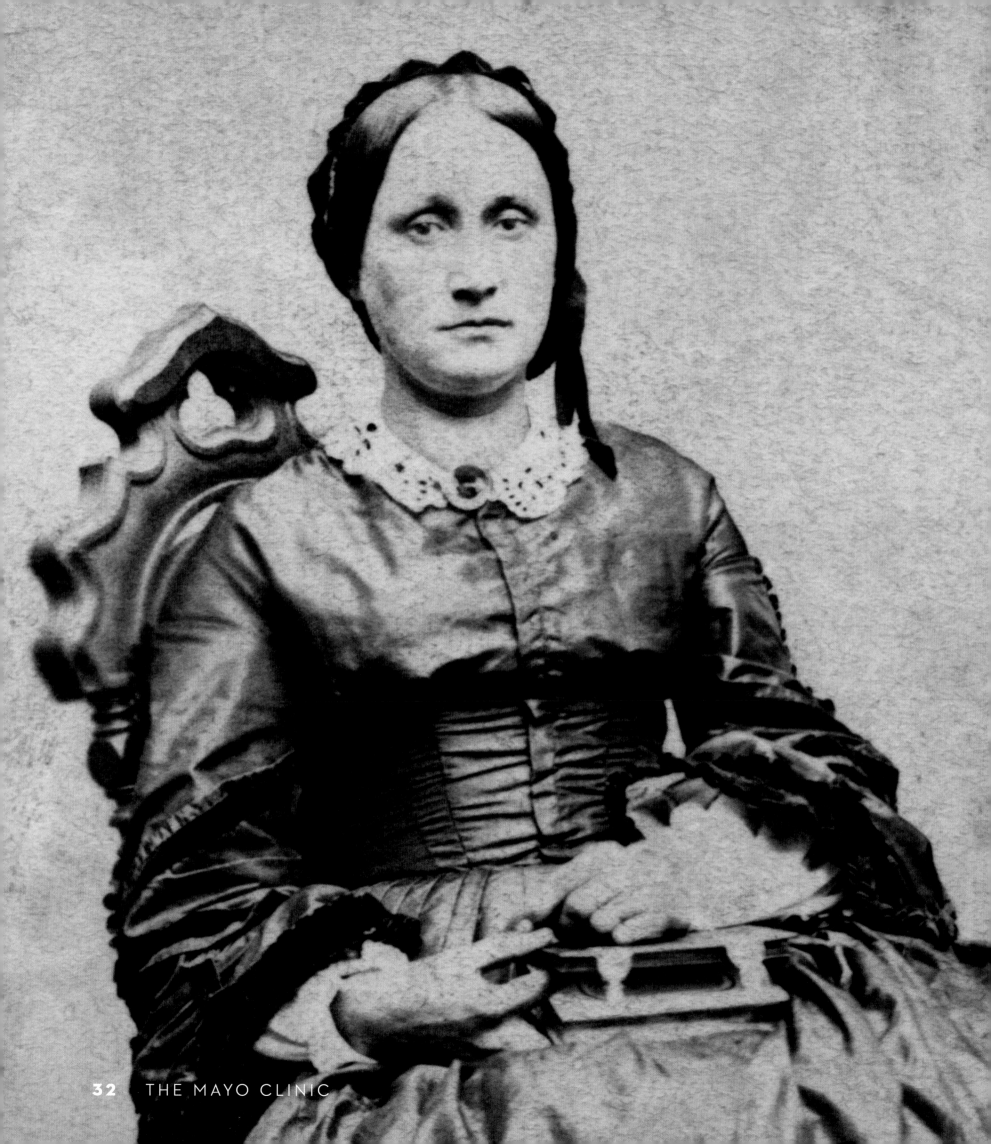

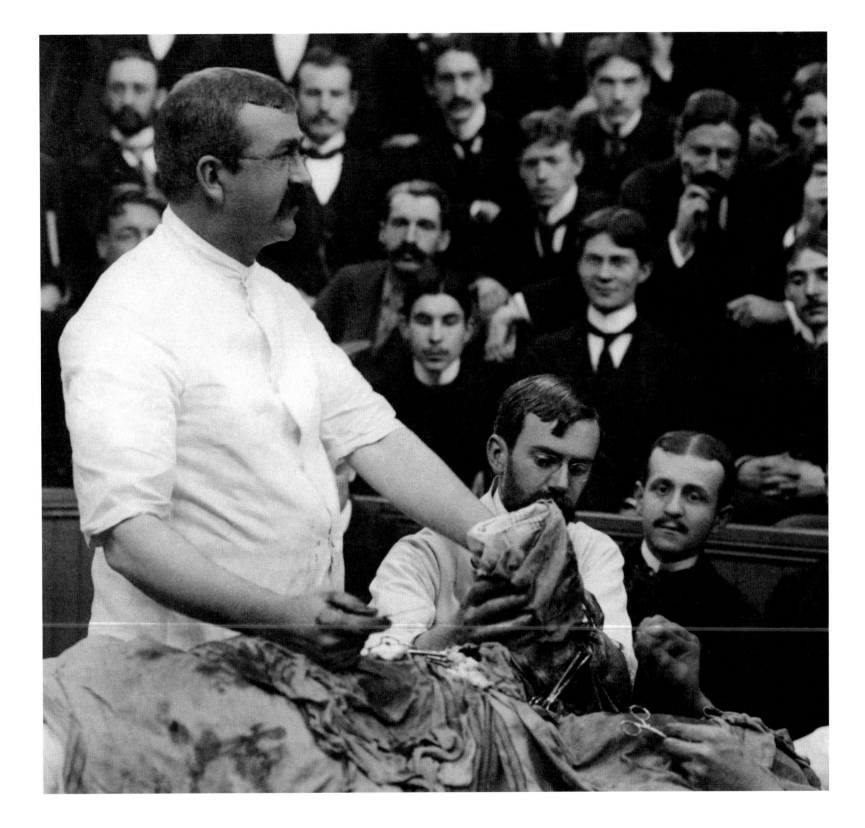

Determined to be a real doctor, W.W. enrolled at the Indiana Medical College. After graduating in 1850, he married 25-year-old Louise Abigail Wright, a strong-willed woman who would become his first assistant. They moved to Lafayette, Indiana, where he opened a practice in a small drugstore. When W.W. contracted malaria, he left the mosquito-infested marshes of Indiana, telling Louise he was going to keep going "until I get well or die."

By the time he arrived in St. Paul, Minnesota, he was well. But wherever he travelled, there were either too many doctors or not enough patients. So for the next ten years, he worked as a surveyor, riverboat pilot, newspaper publisher, and veterinarian.

Opposite: *Louise Mayo*
Next page: *During the Civil War, doctors practiced primitive battlefield medicine.*

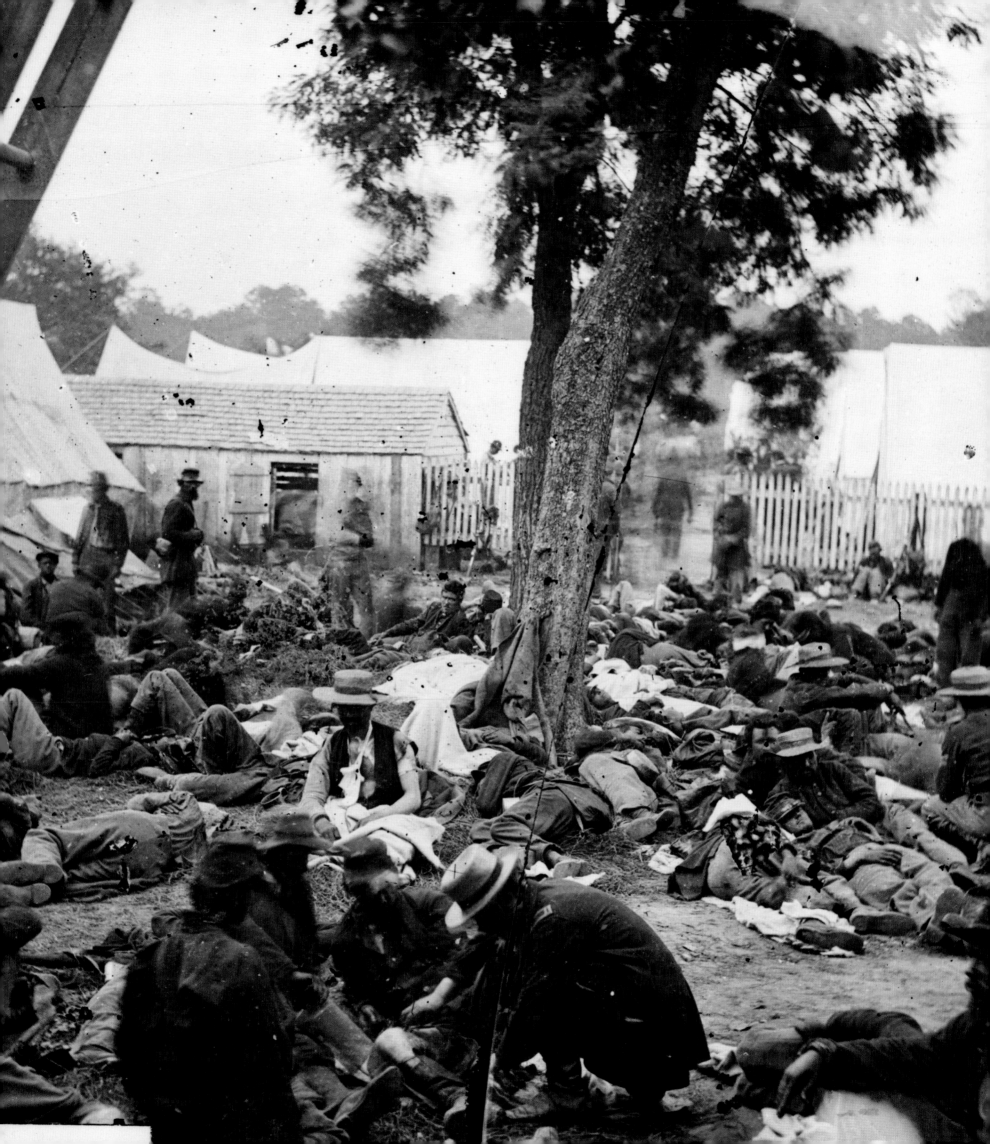

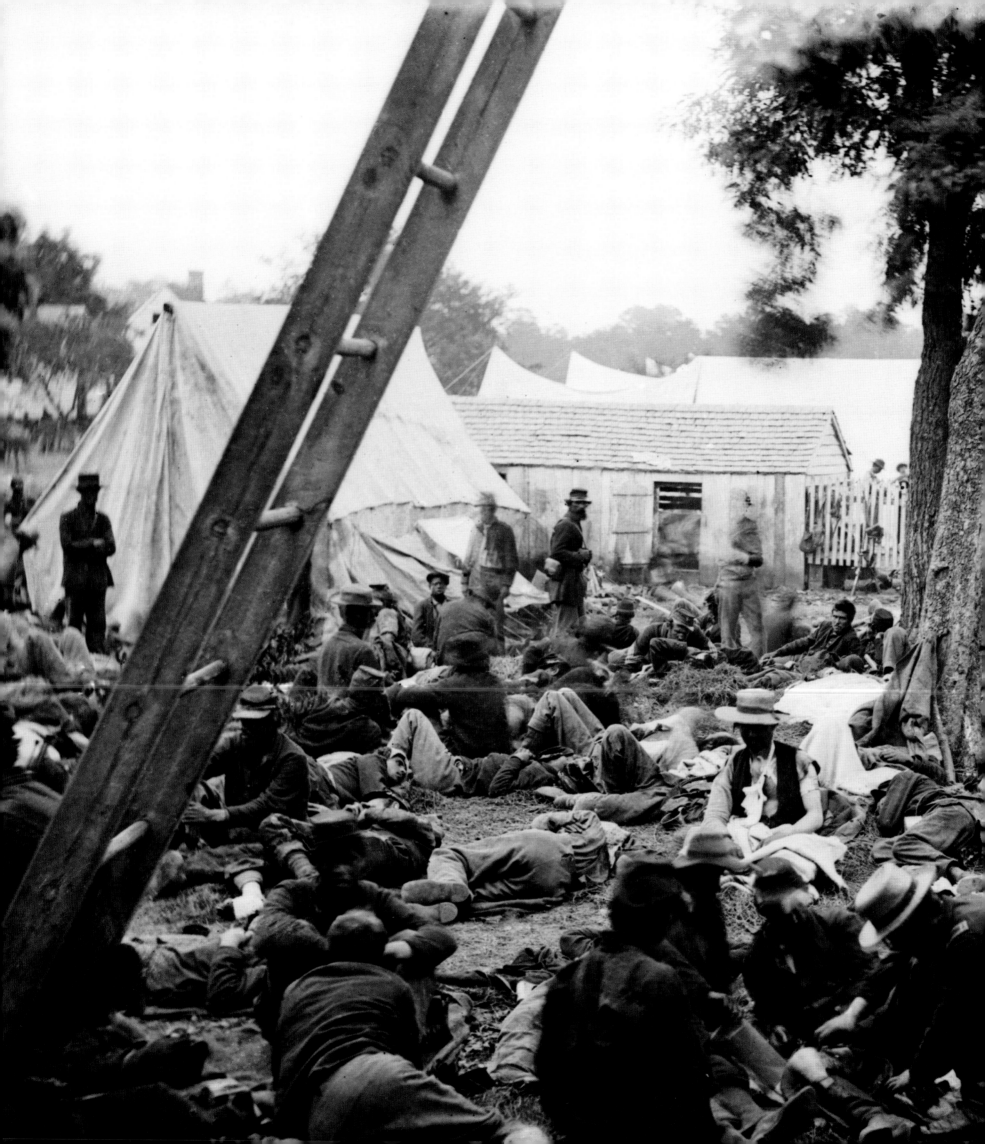

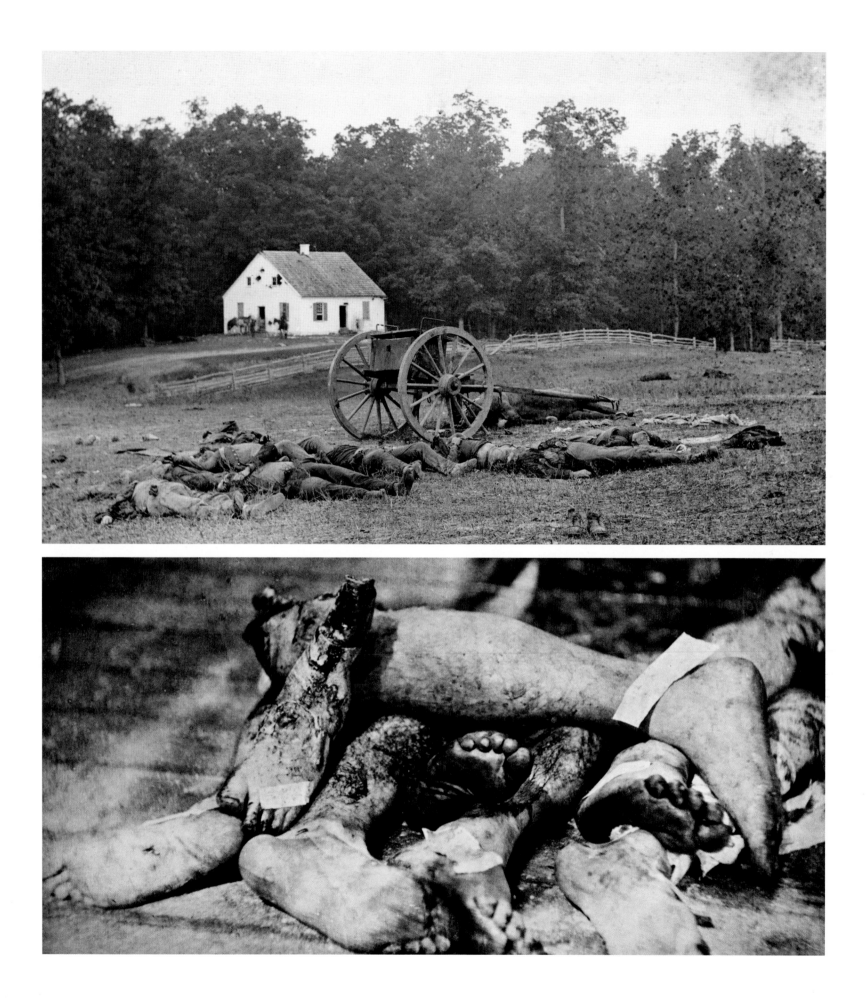

Opposite, top left: *Young Charlie (left) and Will Mayo*

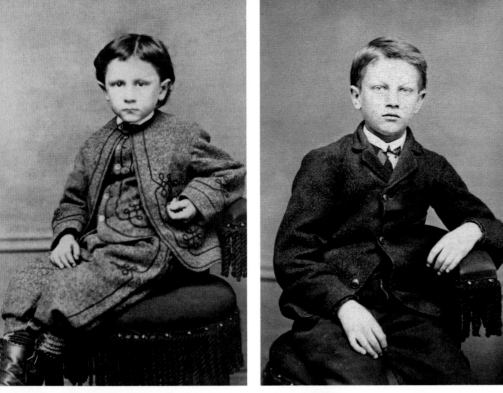

The Civil War brought Mayo's travels to an end. At age 43, W.W. was appointed examining surgeon for a regional enrollment board on the edge of the frontier in Rochester, Minnesota. When Louise and the children caught up with him in January 1864, she told him, "No more. We're not moving again." Although two of their children died in infancy, they eventually had two daughters and two sons, Will and Charlie, whom they would "[raise] in medicine," the boys remembered, "like farm boys on a farm."

While W.W. was trying to determine who was fit to fight for the Union Army, thousands of other doctors were on the battlefield practicing medicine that was almost medieval. Most had never seen a bullet wound, let alone performed surgery. Many sharpened their scalpels on their boots, carried surgical tools in their pockets, and used their own saliva to wet the silk used for sutures.

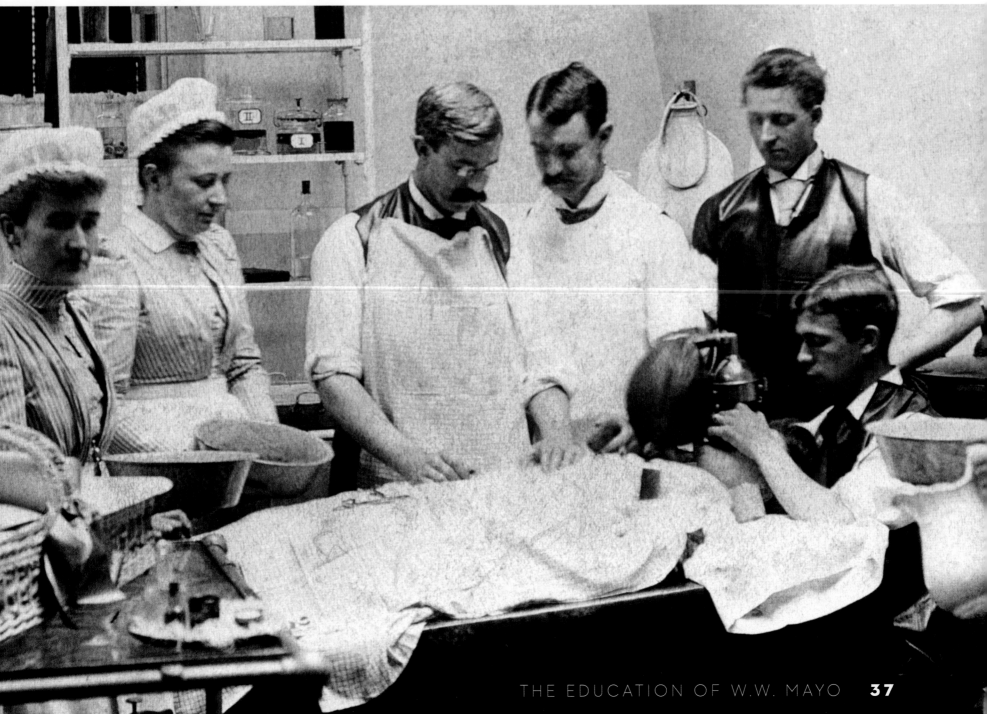

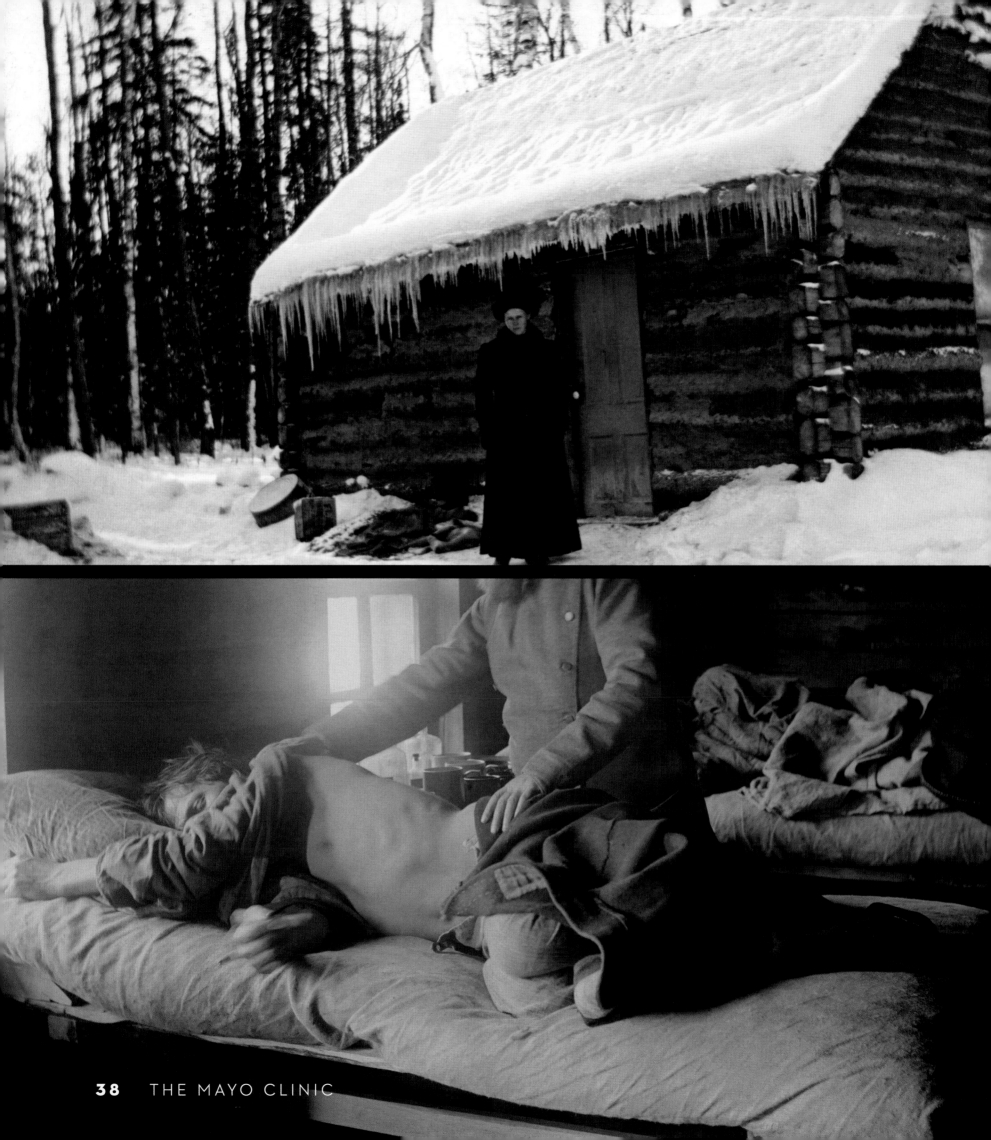

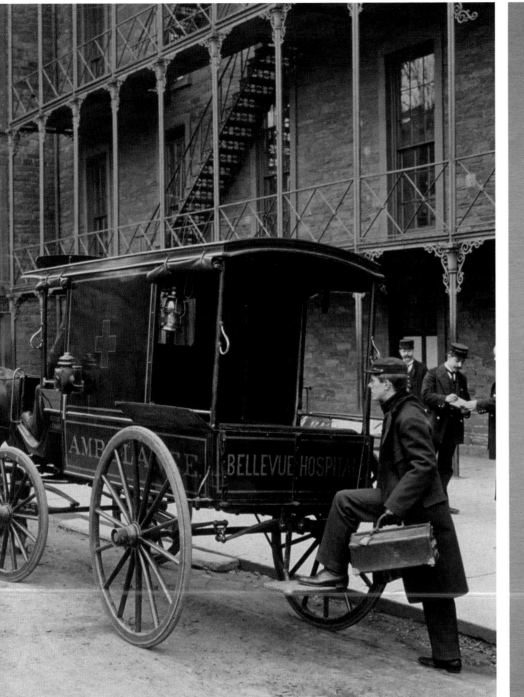

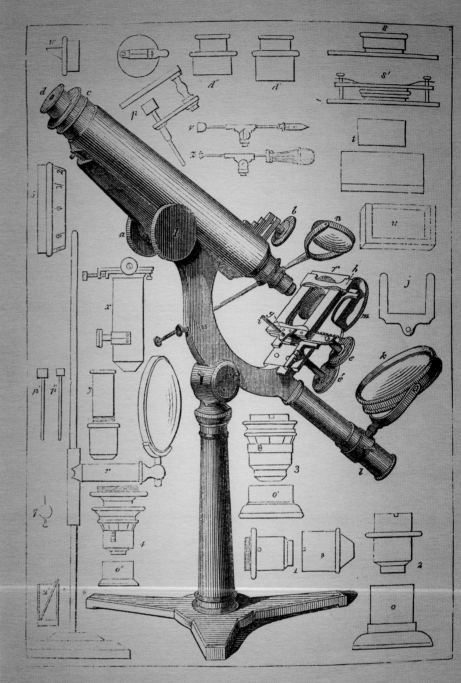

After the war, Mayo began to build a practice in Rochester—and his reputation grew. He usually saw patients at his downtown office, but in an emergency he thought nothing of taking off late at night in the middle of a snowstorm and driving his horse and buggy at breakneck speeds to get to a patient's log or sod home miles away.

He would quickly determine the best place to operate, then proceed to deliver a baby, set the bone of a farmer, or amputate a leg ravaged by gangrene. If the patient was poor, W.W. wouldn't charge him.

He also immersed himself in the latest medical journals, and began contributing his own articles as his expertise increased. Mayo made several return trips to Bellevue Hospital, where he attended lectures, observed operations and autopsies, and marveled at its ambulance corps, the first in New York City. But he was most impressed with an imported German microscope that cost $600—a fortune. When he returned to Rochester, he broached the subject of mortgaging their house to pay for the new instrument. Louise was loath to take on any more debt, but she finally said, "If it's of use to the people...let's do it."

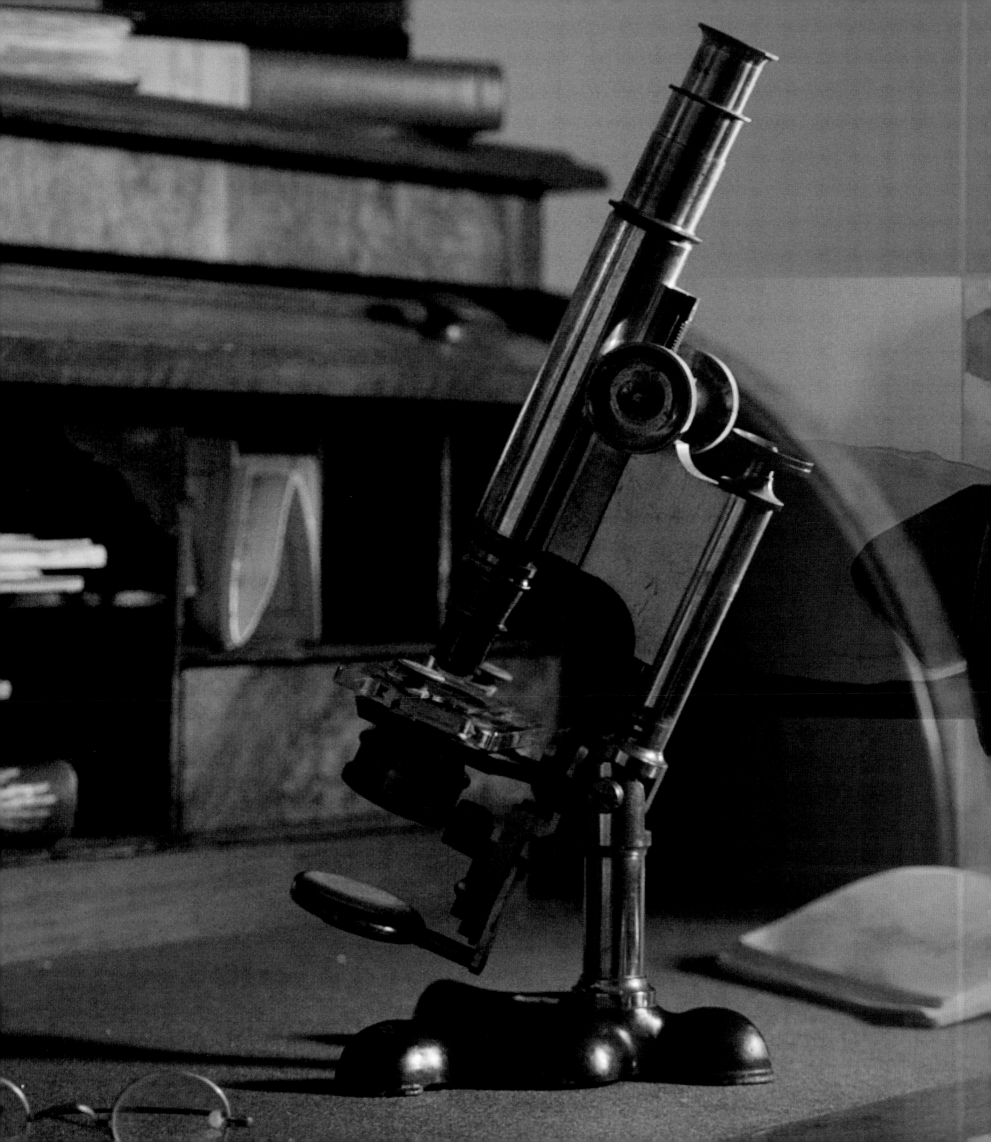

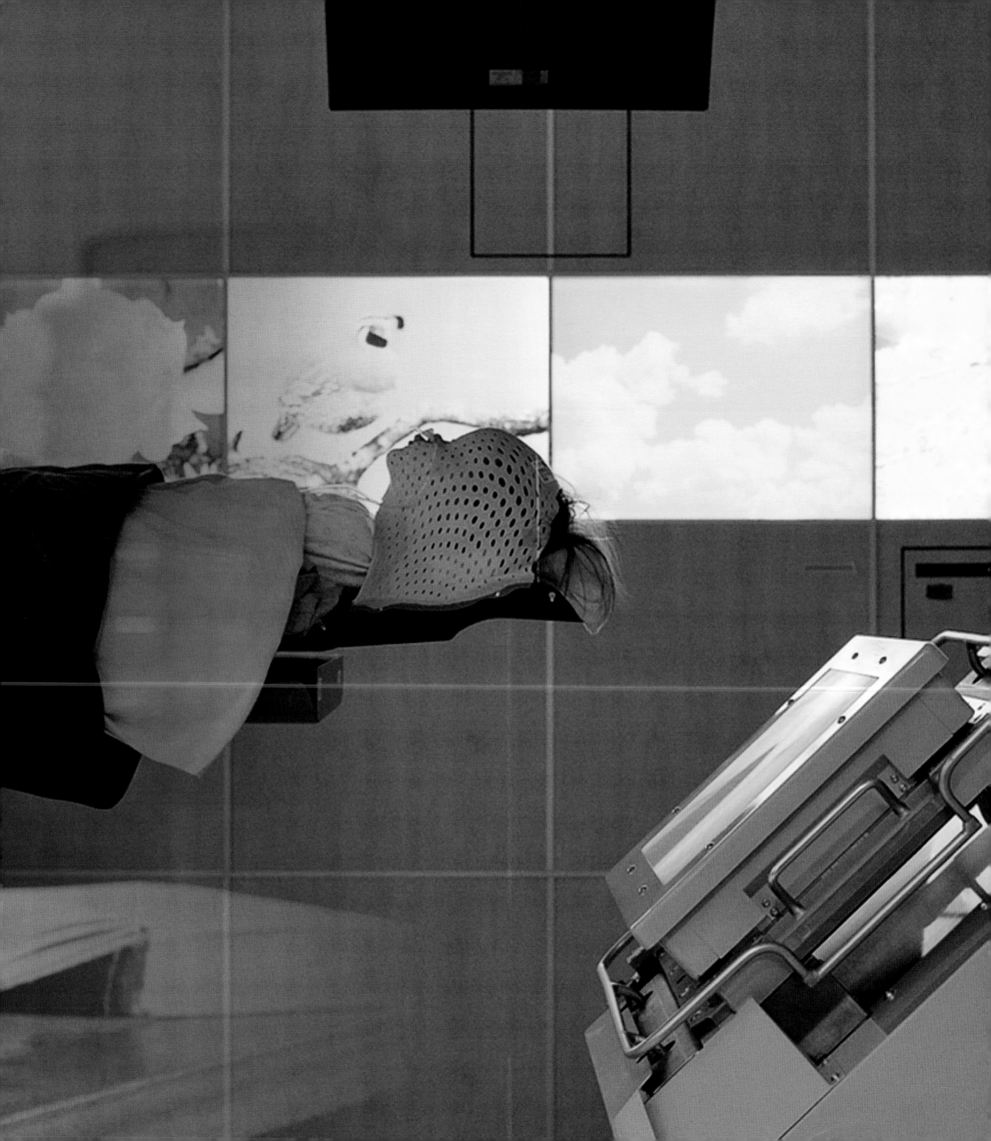

DIAGNOSIS: BRAIN CANCER

Alyssa Feenstra (Salt Lake City, UT): This doctor comes in and he pulls the chair over to the bedside, sits down, and says, "There's no easy way to say this, but your daughter has a mass in her brain." The neurosurgeons in Salt Lake City did an amazing job. But, for me, I always knew that it wasn't just surgery.

Christopher Feenstra (Salt Lake City, UT): The proton beam—radiation—is what brought us out to Mayo Clinic. I said that I would go to India if that was the best place my kid could be. Mayo Clinic is my India. Things happen in life. People die. Mayo Clinic can't save everybody. It's not magic. And blasting my child's head for six weeks while she's trying to develop these cognitive and extremely important pathways in her brain, that's just ludicrous. But when we got to Mayo Clinic and met with Dr. Keole, he said, "You know what? I can't promise you anything, but we're going to have a strategic plan on how to outmaneuver whatever adversary you're looking at." That was different; that was a big difference.

Mayo Clinic didn't happen out of thin air. And I know Mayo Clinic has a reputation, but I didn't understand what that was. I didn't get it until Abigail got brain cancer. Health care is a customer service–based experience. And I hate using the term *customer service* because it makes it sound like I'm at Applebee's, about to tip the waitress. We had a lot of different experiences with different health care across the nation. What blew me away about the Mayo experience was that it showed me what was lacking in other places.

Sameer Keole, M.D. (Mayo Clinic oncologist): In Abby's case, we want to treat the cavity where the tumor has been resected. X-ray therapy—which is what 99.5 percent of centers in this country use—goes in through the patient and out of the patient, and exits on the other side. Proton therapy is a charged particle. It will go a set distance in tissue, then stops on a dime, and literally all the energy gets released right at that point. And that's how we kill the cancer. We should be able to completely spare that area of the brain that the most important part of learning in a child, so we reduce the long-term complications. We recognize there's a huge controversy over price. Proton therapy is a $360 million investment by Mayo Clinic. Cost is an important topic, especially in today's health economics environment, where our health-care costs are spiraling. But if protons could be built and operated for the same exact cost as X-ray therapy, we wouldn't be having this discussion. So at Mayo Clinic we decided to charge exactly the same for proton therapy as we do for X-ray therapy. We are going to eat this cost.

AF: We go home from treatment and she is a normal 18-month-old. We're coming to an end. And I couldn't have asked for anything better for her. I've never experienced health care in a team like Abigail has. There's hope for her future.

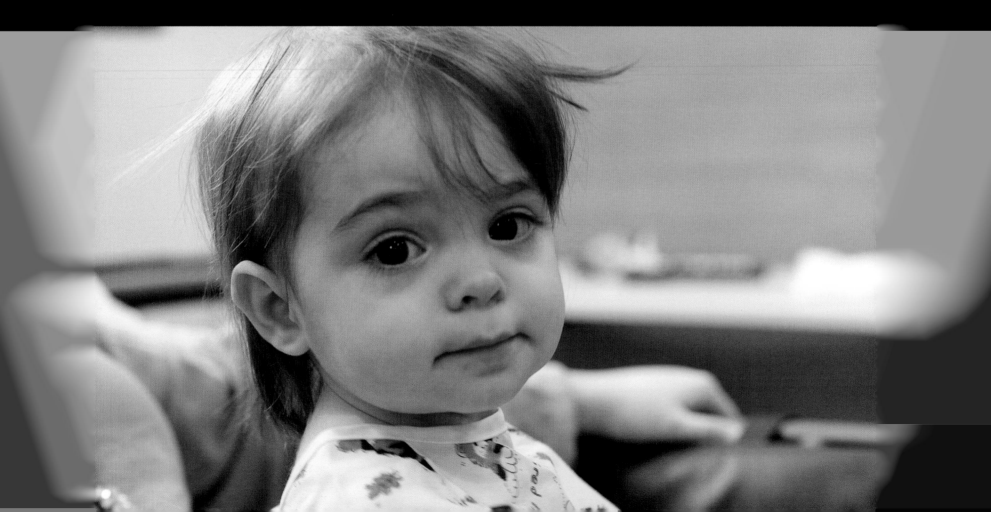

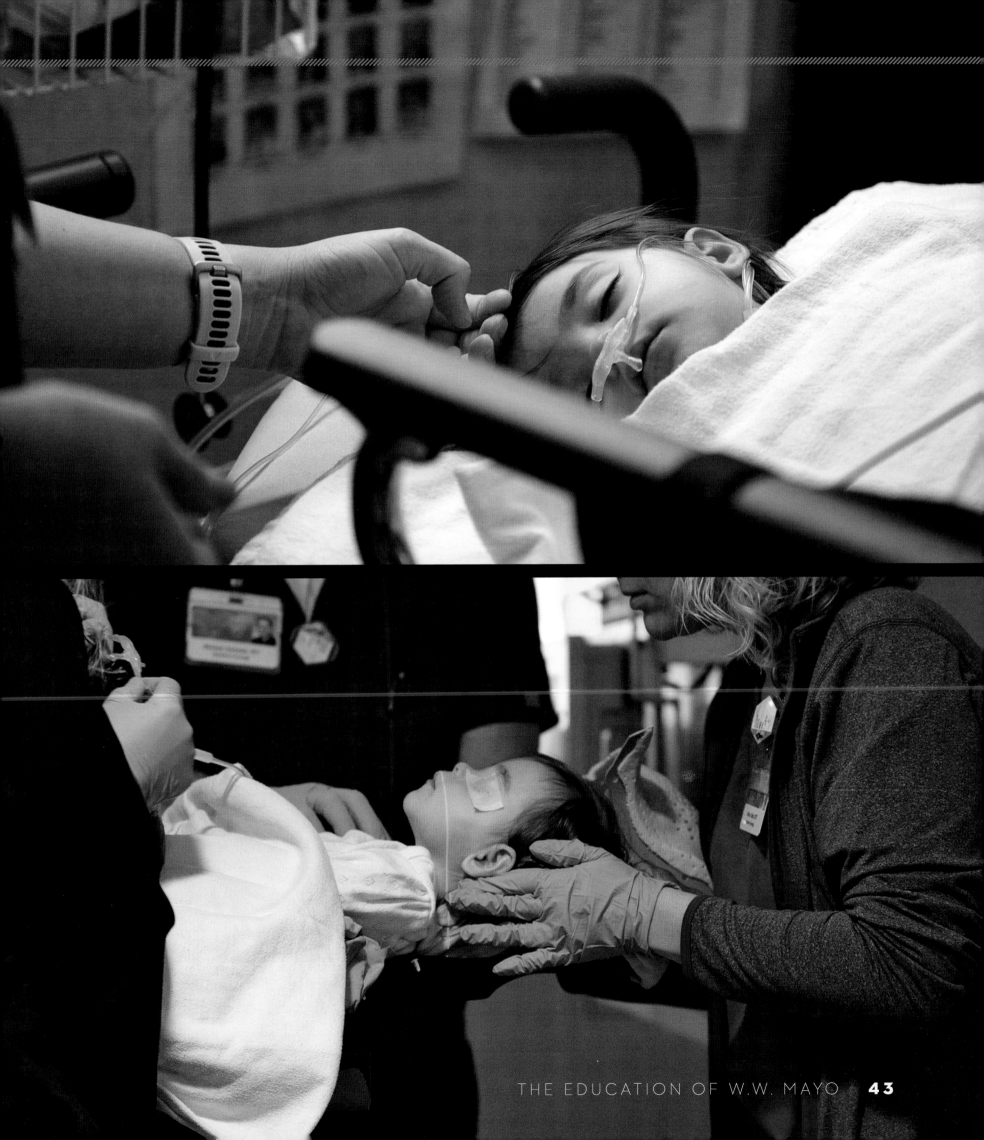

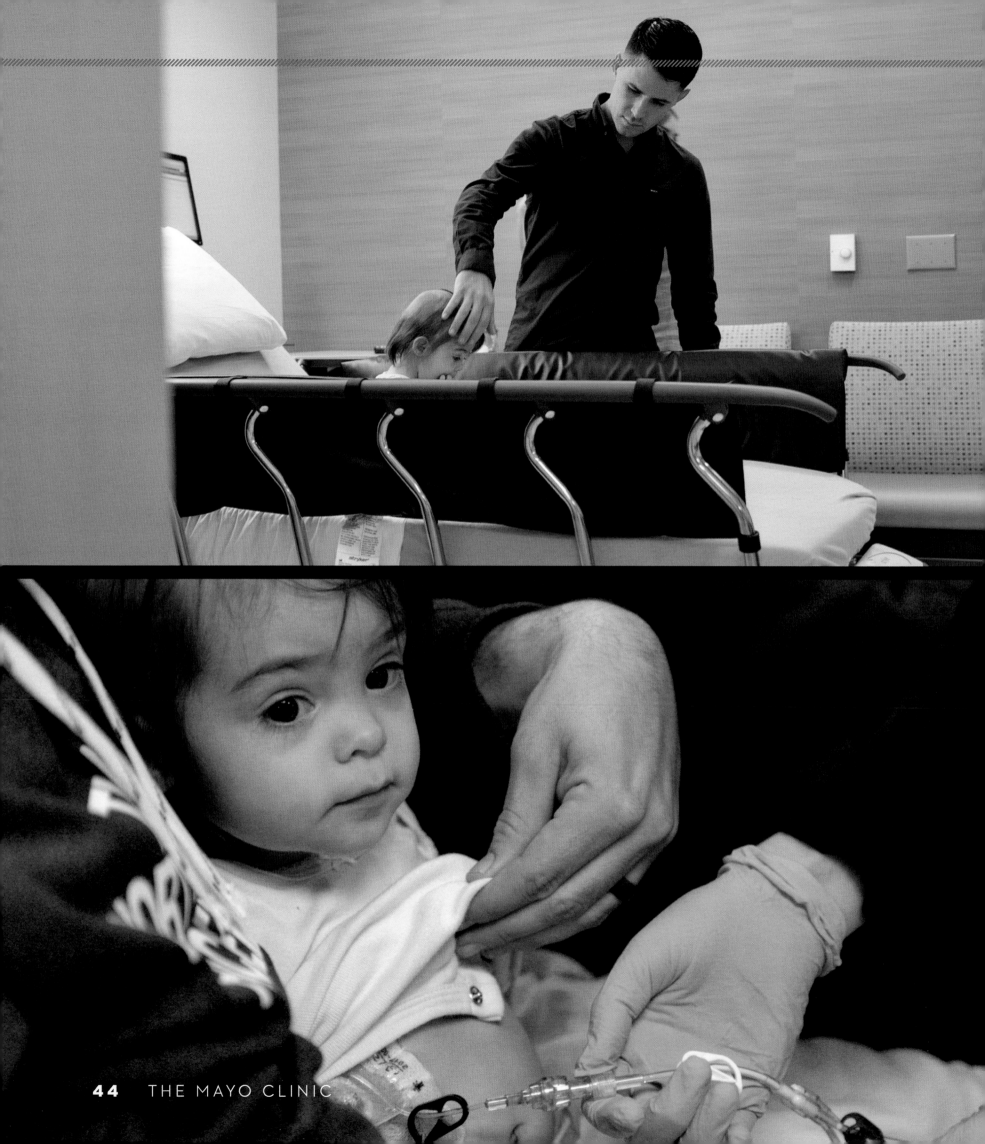

The health-care system has gone a bit overboard by assuming that consumerism and competition alone will somehow clean up everything, and they haven't. There's a great deal of frustration because of the way health insurance is organized. But the idealism is still there. I hope the age of consumerism in health care will be followed by an age of idealism during which organizations feel that they have an obligation to do the very best no matter what the cost.

—ROSEMARY A. STEVENS, PH.D., MEDICAL HISTORIAN, WEILL CORNELL MEDICINE

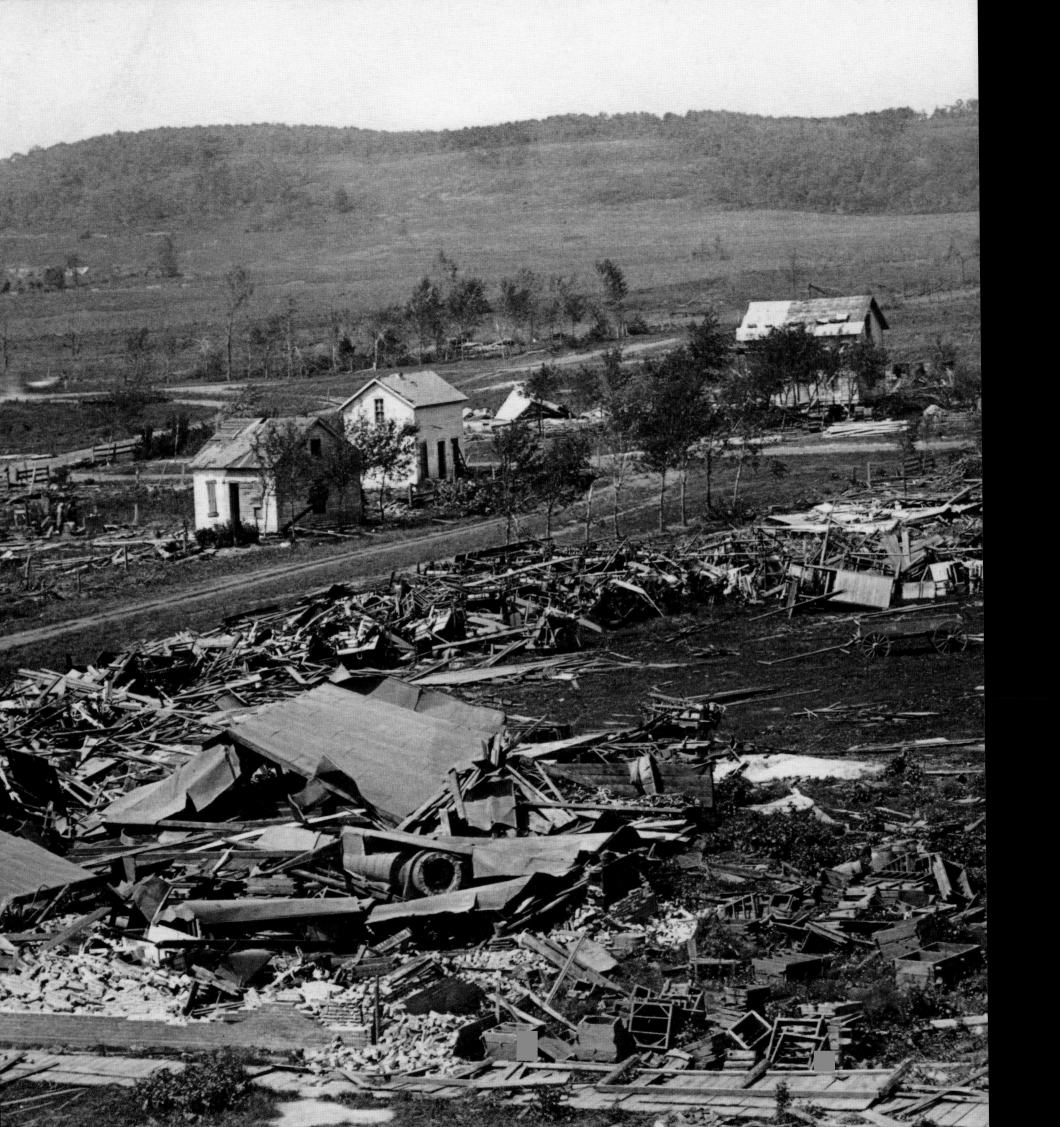

CHAPTER TWO

A TORNADO AND A HANDSHAKE

With our faith and hope and energy, it will succeed.

—MOTHER ALFRED MOES

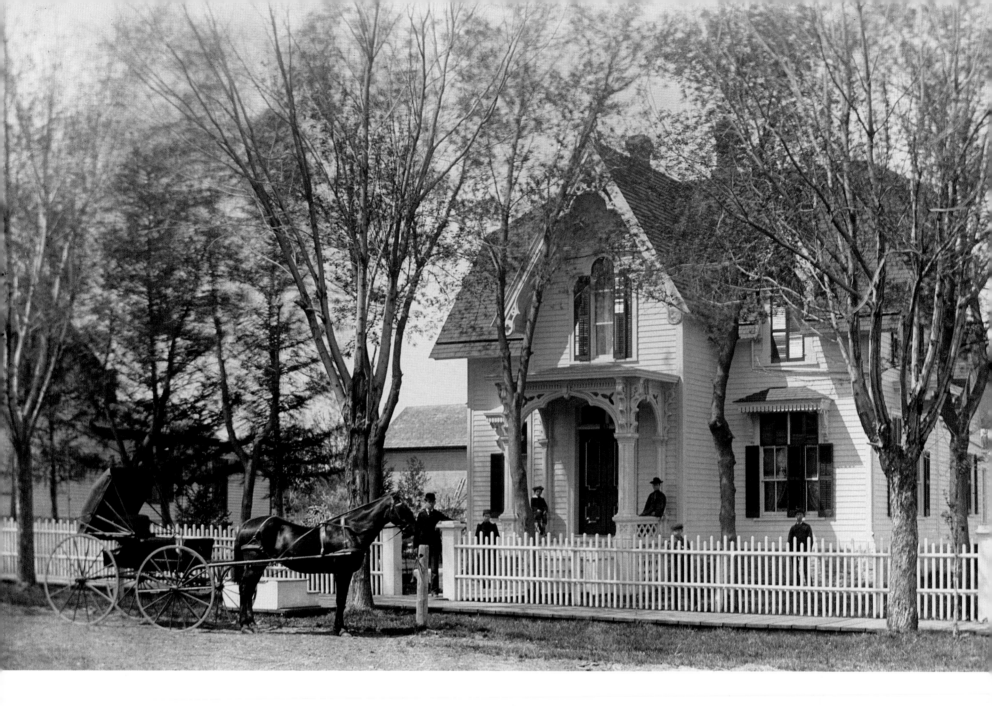

From the time they were little boys, when W.W. went to visit patients in the country, Will and Charlie went along with their father in the buggy. This buggy became a traveling schoolroom for the boys. He encouraged the boys to observe and then he would pose problems.

—JUDITH HARTZELL, HISTORIAN AND AUTHOR, ROCHESTER, IN

Will and Charlie began their medical careers sweeping floors and washing windows in their father's office. Eventually, he took them on house calls and let them help care for patients. At day's end, they sat together and discussed what they had seen. Louise also helped by assisting at surgeries, treating injuries, and counseling patients who showed up when her husband was away. As Charlie said, "The biggest thing Will and I ever did was to pick the father and mother we had." Both boys went to medical school—the older Will to the University of Michigan, and Charlie at Northwestern.

More than twenty people died in the tornado that swept through Rochester that summer day in 1883, and dozens more were injured. The Sisters of Saint Francis did what they could to help, but afterward Mother Alfred knew they could have done more. Then she had her vision of building a hospital that would, she insisted, be open to "all sick persons regardless of their color, sex, financial status, or professed religion."

The Rochester Post.

EXTRA.

VOL. XIV.   NO. 37

THE CYCLONE

OLMSTED COUNTY SUFFERS SEVERELY FROM THE STORM.

A Number of Persons Killed and Injured.

blown to pieces. Mrs. Jones was struck with a large timber across the forehead and seriously injured. Her recovery is considered doubtful.

The barn of Thos. Jones, in section 14, Kalmar, was unroofed.

From H. A. Eckholdt, Judge Start, F. B. Kellogg, and A. L. Gove, who went out by the river road directly north eight miles, we learn the following particulars:

At John Klee's house the wing was blown to pieces and scattered over the country. The families of D. Sonnenburg and G. Bodelske had taken

corners was entirely demolished, not a brick being left standing.

John Hoffman's barn, near Douglass, was blown to pieces.

The houses of M. Kolbe and M. Beneke were blown to pieces.

O. R. Pease, who lives near the poor farm, in the town of Rochester, had a new hay shed 64 feet long, lifted bodily and thrown on top of his cow shed, injuring it considerably.

The town of Elgin, in Wabasha county, was completely wrecked, but one building, the railroad elevator, being left standing. One lady, a p

one could be found that could be used. Mr. Harvey's mother, an elderly lady, was nearly buried in the ruins of the stone building. Messrs. Harvey estimate their loss at $3,000. The family in the frame building escaped by going into the cellar.

A barn on the farm of Mr. F. Beneke was blown away.

Mr. E. T. Dodge's house was moved 85 feet from the foundation; crops injured, and barn demolished.

The residence and barn of Mr. Sumner Snow was torn to pieces. His household furniture and dishes were

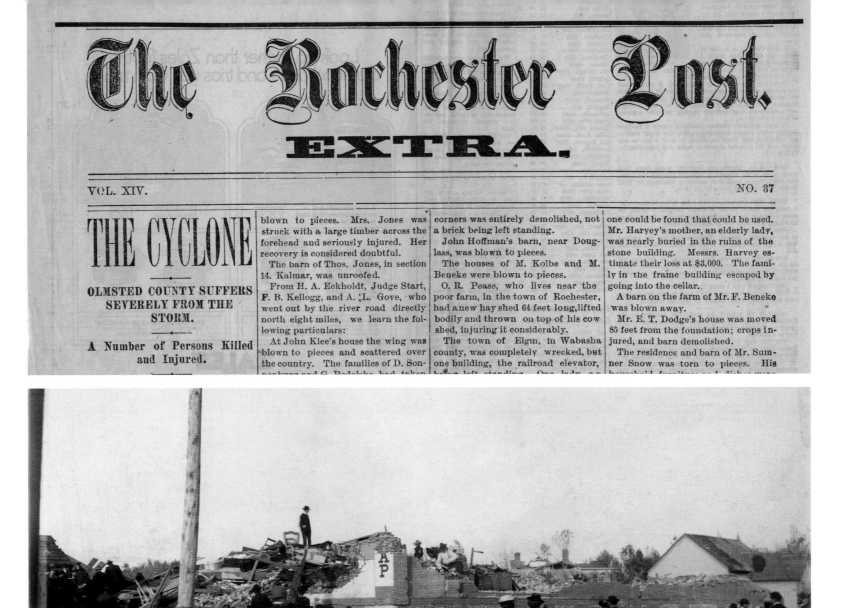

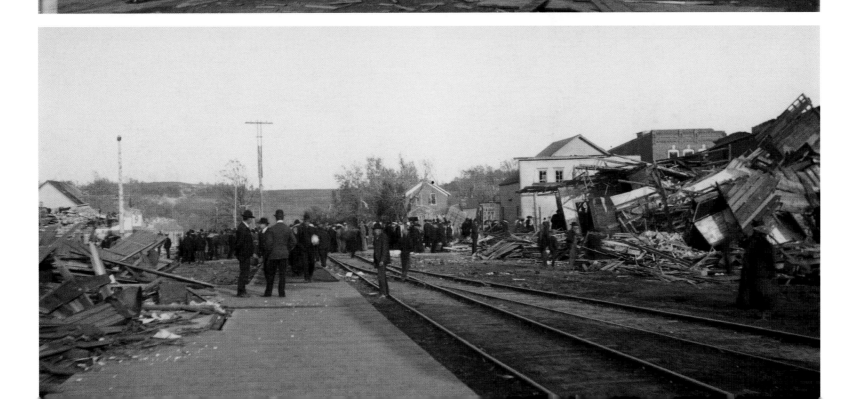

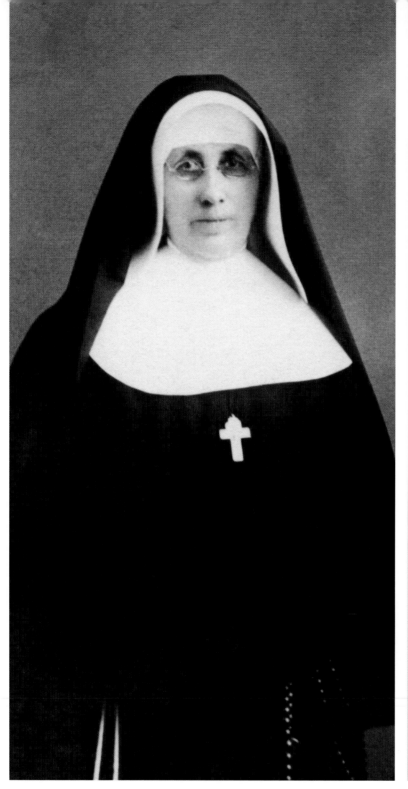
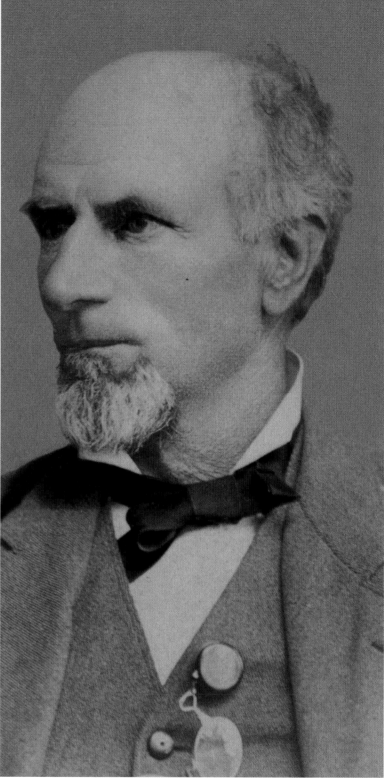

Mother Alfred was a 53-year-old nun who believed "the cause of suffering humanity knows no religion." Doctor Mayo was a 64-year-old agnostic who, a newspaperman remembered, "defended Darwin by the hour." Both were stubborn and impetuous—and driven by a desire to serve.

Mayo was certain Mother Alfred would be unable to raise the money. She could buy the land she wanted just west of town for $2,000, but the building would cost at least $40,000. He reluctantly agreed that if she succeeded in securing the funds, he would lead its medical staff and perform all his surgeries there while still running his practice downtown.

He thought, "There's no way they're going to raise $40,000." And she was convinced—she knew the Sisters would raise that money, and she would hold him to that.

—SISTER TIERNEY TRUEMAN, ORDER OF SAINT FRANCIS, ROCHESTER, MN

Above: Mother Alfred and W.W.

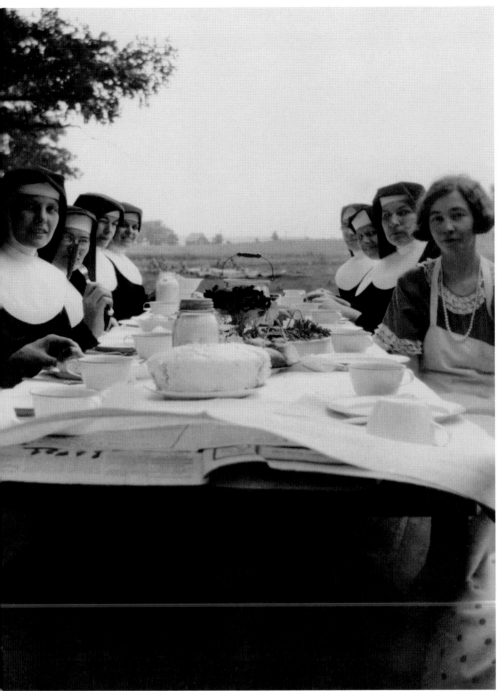

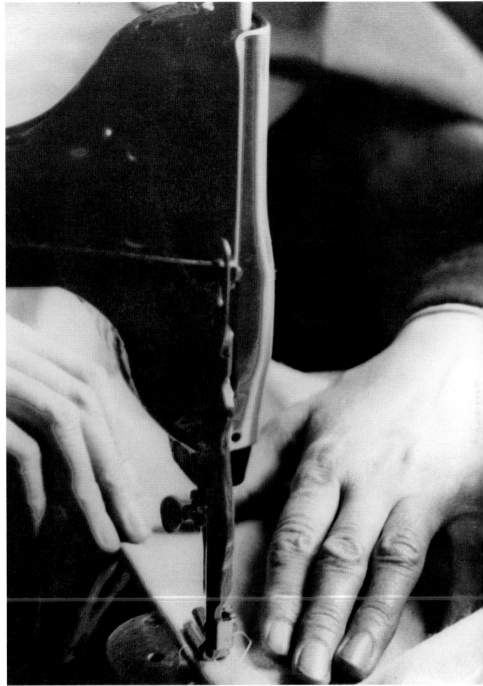

Mother Alfred and William Worrall never drew up any legal documents. Their word and that handshake meant everything.

—RENEE ZIEMER,
MAYO CLINIC HISTORIAN

They shook on it. For the next 100 years, every agreement between Mayo Clinic and the Sisters of Saint Francis would be made that way.

Mother Alfred and the nuns set to work. They saved every penny they could from tuitions at their schools. They also gave music lessons, embroidered linens, chopped their own wood, made pillowcases out of flour sacks, and ate the simplest of meals. After five long years, construction finally began in August 1888.

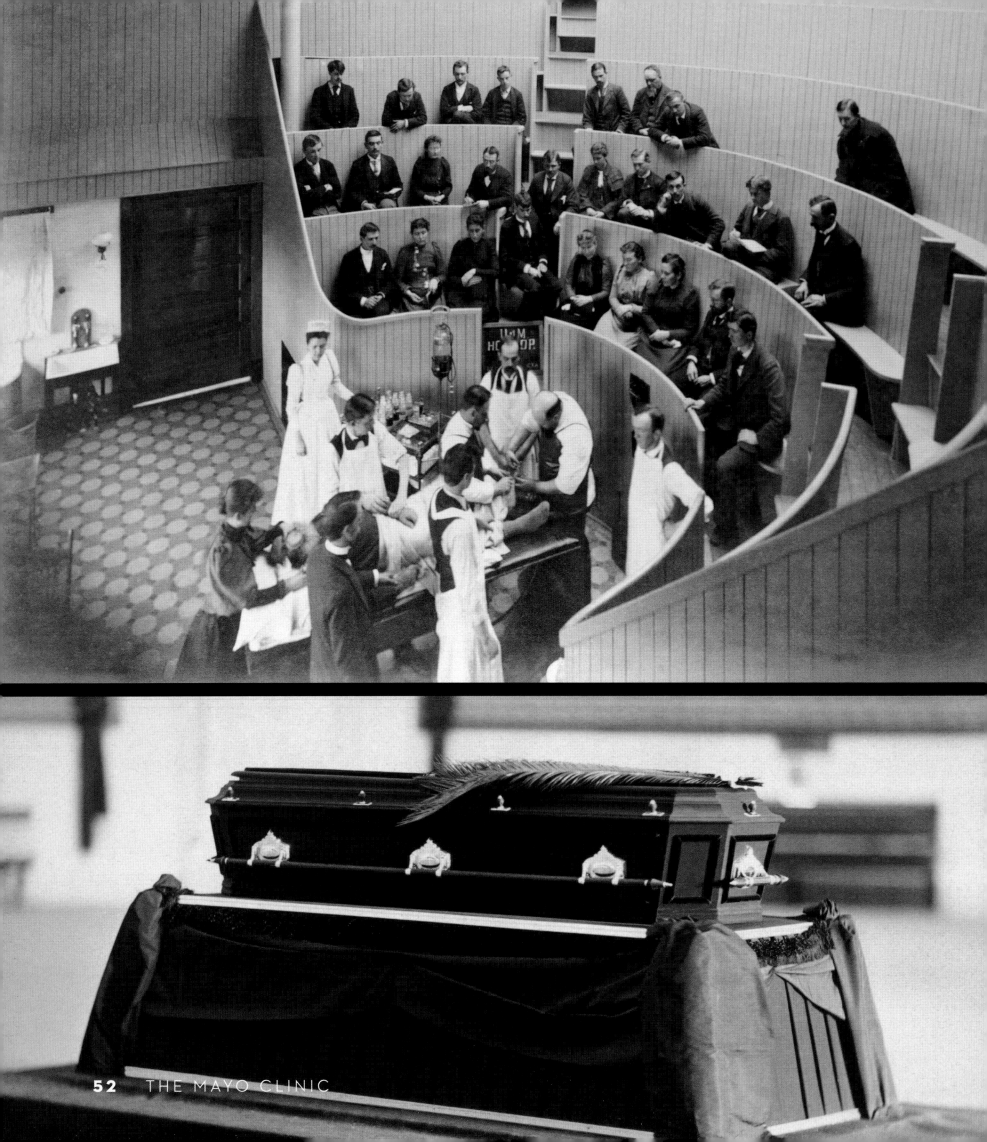

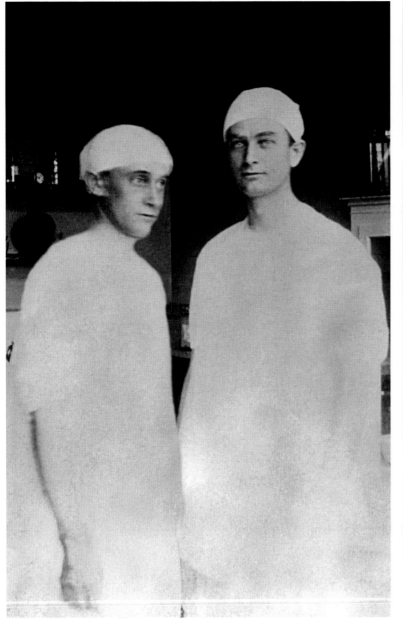

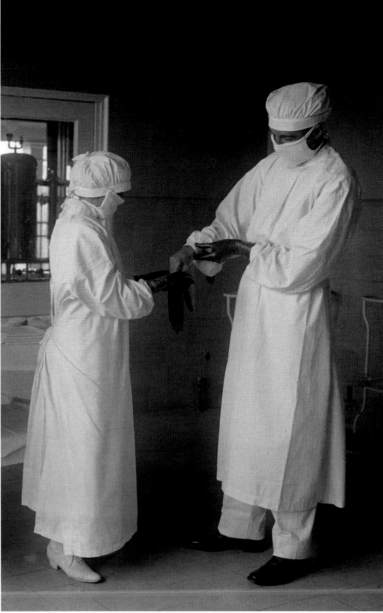

Meanwhile, Will and Charlie began to play a major role in their father's practice. They had become passionate advocates for a new procedure developed by a Scottish surgeon named Joseph Lister, based on the theory that germs cause infections.

Most American doctors were skeptical of this idea. (In 1881, President James A. Garfield had died not from his would-be assassin's bullet, but because of his doctors' filthy, unwashed hands.) But the Mayos were convinced. They designed and equipped the operating rooms for the new hospital specifically to take advantage of the latest innovations in sterilization.

> There was an air of curiosity, an imagination, all the way from the beginning of the history of the Clinic, looking for new methods, new science, new techniques. They were forward looking and conservative at the same time.
>
> **—ROSEMARY A. STEVENS, PH.D., MEDICAL HISTORIAN, WEILL CORNELL MEDICINE**

Opposite, below: *President Garfield's casket*
Top left: *Dr. Charlie (left) and Dr. Will*

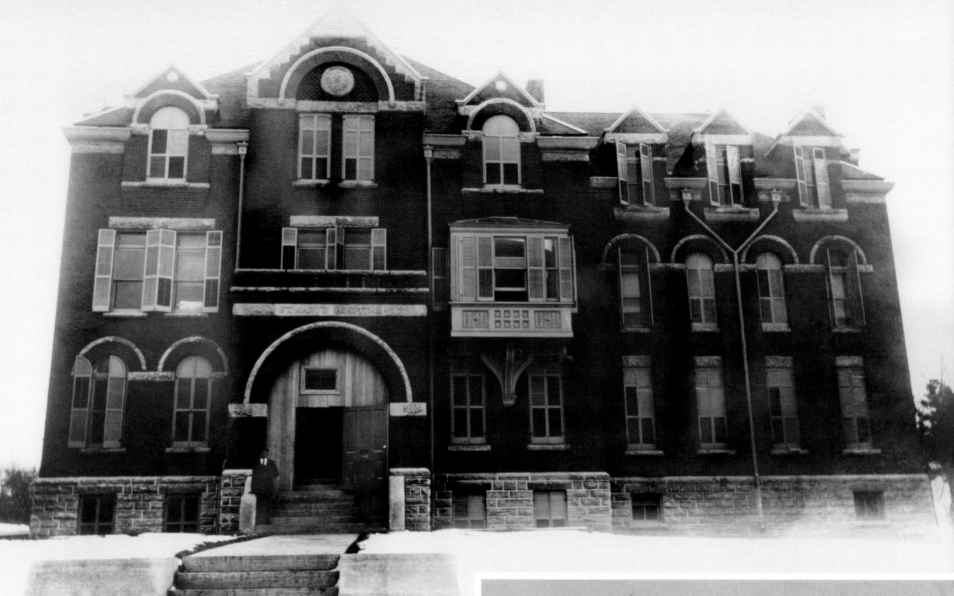

On September 30, 1889, the day before the new facility officially opened, the Mayo brothers performed eye surgery on a man from Olmsted County. He was the very first patient admitted to Rochester's brand-new hospital. It was called Saint Marys.

So, with no more fanfare than just a blessing, the hospital was open, a patient was admitted and had surgery, and the only thing it says about him is that he got well and went home.

—SISTER GENEROSE GERVAIS, ORDER OF SAINT FRANCIS, ROCHESTER, MN

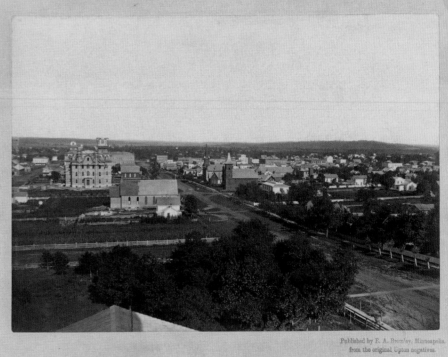

Published by E. A. Bromley, Minneapolis.
from the original Upton negatives.

ROCHESTER,
MINNESOTA 1887.

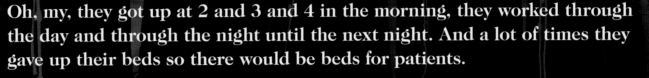

Oh, my, they got up at 2 and 3 and 4 in the morning, they worked through the day and through the night until the next night. And a lot of times they gave up their beds so there would be beds for patients.

—SISTER LAUREN WEINANDT, ORDER OF SAINT FRANCIS, ROCHESTER, MN

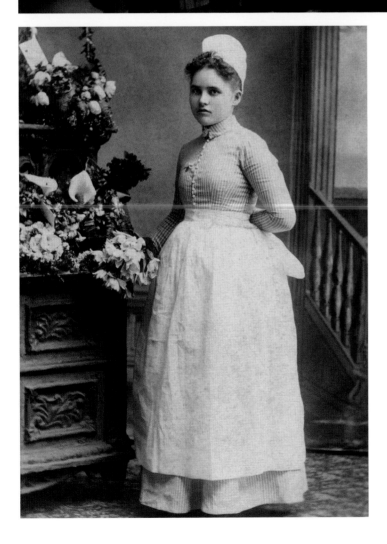

From the outside, Saint Marys was an impressive, modern-looking, three-story brick building. But inside, the Sisters who were responsible for taking care of the patients couldn't have asked for a harder test of their faith. They did the nursing, the laundry, the cooking, the cleaning. They did everything.

The nuns who lived and worked at Saint Marys had trained as teachers, not nurses. Edith Graham, a Rochester native who had completed nursing school, joined the Mayos' downtown practice on Third Street. But she ended up spending most of her time a mile away at Saint Marys, where she took care of patients and shared her knowledge with the Sisters.

Of the first 400 surgeries performed by the Mayos at Saint Marys Hospital, only two patients died.

I have no idea how the Sisters took care of patients with so little, but they made a way. And that's one thing about being a nurse: you make a way out of no way.

—QUIANA DEBRILL, L.P.N., MAYO CLINIC

Bottom: Edith Graham

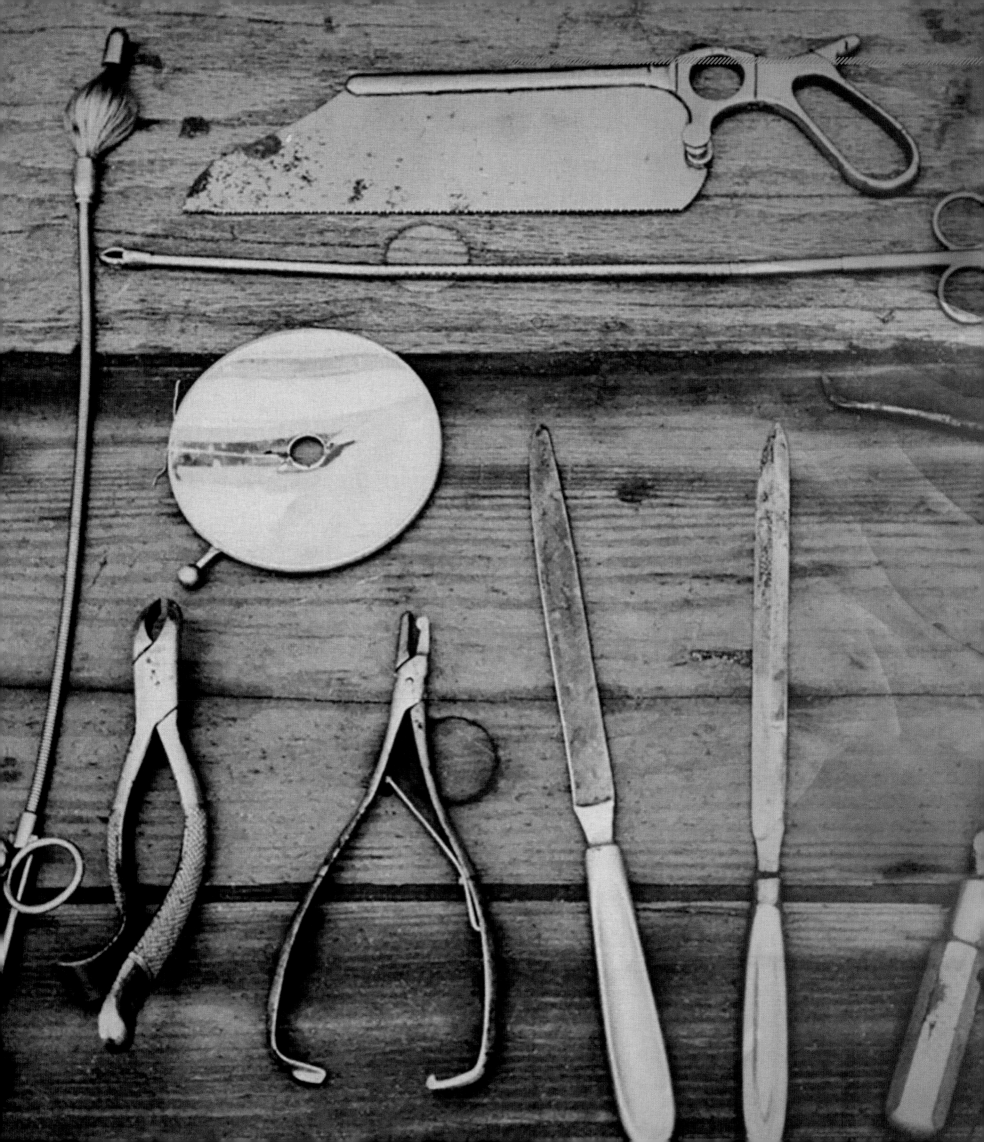

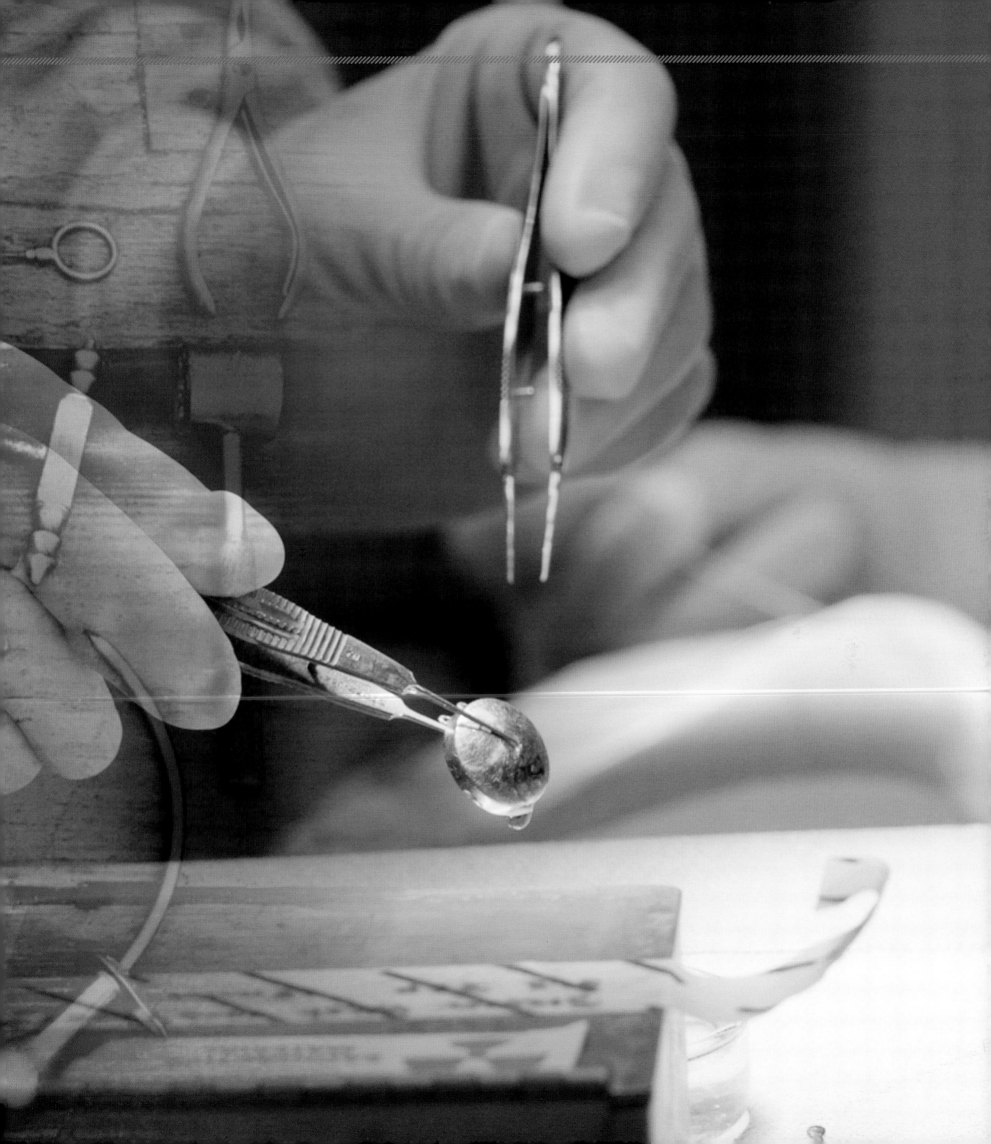

DIAGNOSIS: CANCER OF THE EYE

ALICEN BUCK (Minot, ND): Two months before I went to the Mayo Clinic, I started noticing that I had double vision, so I scheduled an appointment to see the ophthalmologist. As soon as they said something about melanoma, we just were in shock. Because all you think about is the worst: *Will I be able to stay pregnant?*

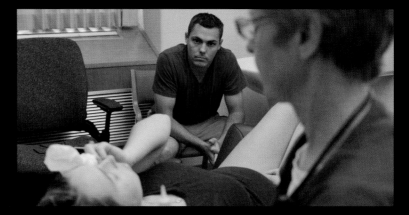

JOSE PULIDO, M.D. (Mayo Clinic surgical ophthalmologist): The same factors that were letting her baby grow were allowing the cancer cells to grow as well. I've seen these patients who are pregnant with melanomas; their cancer cells grow exuberantly.

AB: Dr. Pulido basically sat down and told me that my life was at risk and I really needed to think about terminating. That was very hard to hear. What came in my head was, *Is there another way? Can you just take my eye, please? Just don't take my baby.* He told us that he was good with the eyes, not with the babies. But he already had the appointment scheduled with the OB.

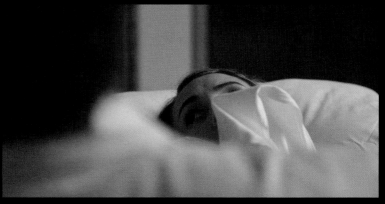

MARI CHARISSE TRINIDAD, M.D. (Mayo Clinic obstetrician and gynecologist): These are hard conversations to have. Whenever you have a mother with a high-risk medical condition, you need to have different providers with different areas of expertise. A lot of data around the impact of pregnancy on melanomas is conflicting. At that point, options were still available for her despite the pregnancy. But the risk of metastases is there. Melanoma is actually one of the most common cancers that can spread, even to the fetus. We reviewed what she wanted to do, and she was very clear that she did not want to proceed with elective termination.

JP: For her, we used a plaque, which looks like a bottle cap. You put radioactive seeds within it, and then you sew this on the eye, so the gold doesn't allow the radiation to come anywhere but into the eye. Sometimes I deal with people who die. I feel that the only way that I can give them hope is if I know in my heart of hearts I'm trying to push the boundaries. After that it was kind of a wait-and-see situation to see whether the melanoma cells were responsive.

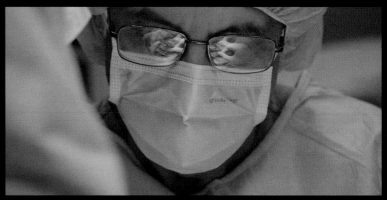

Four months later

AB: We came to find out about my melanoma and see if it shrank.

JP: So, there's nothing in the liver, and the chest X-ray is fine as well. And the tumor is starting to shrink.

AB: My radiation worked! And so the melanoma is shrinking; it's basically dead now, which is very nice.

JP: It's pretty interesting that the first case done at Saint Marys was removal of an eye for an eye cancer.

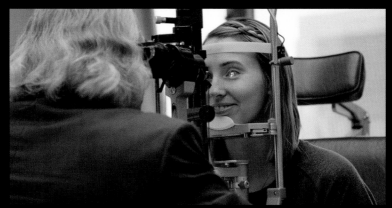

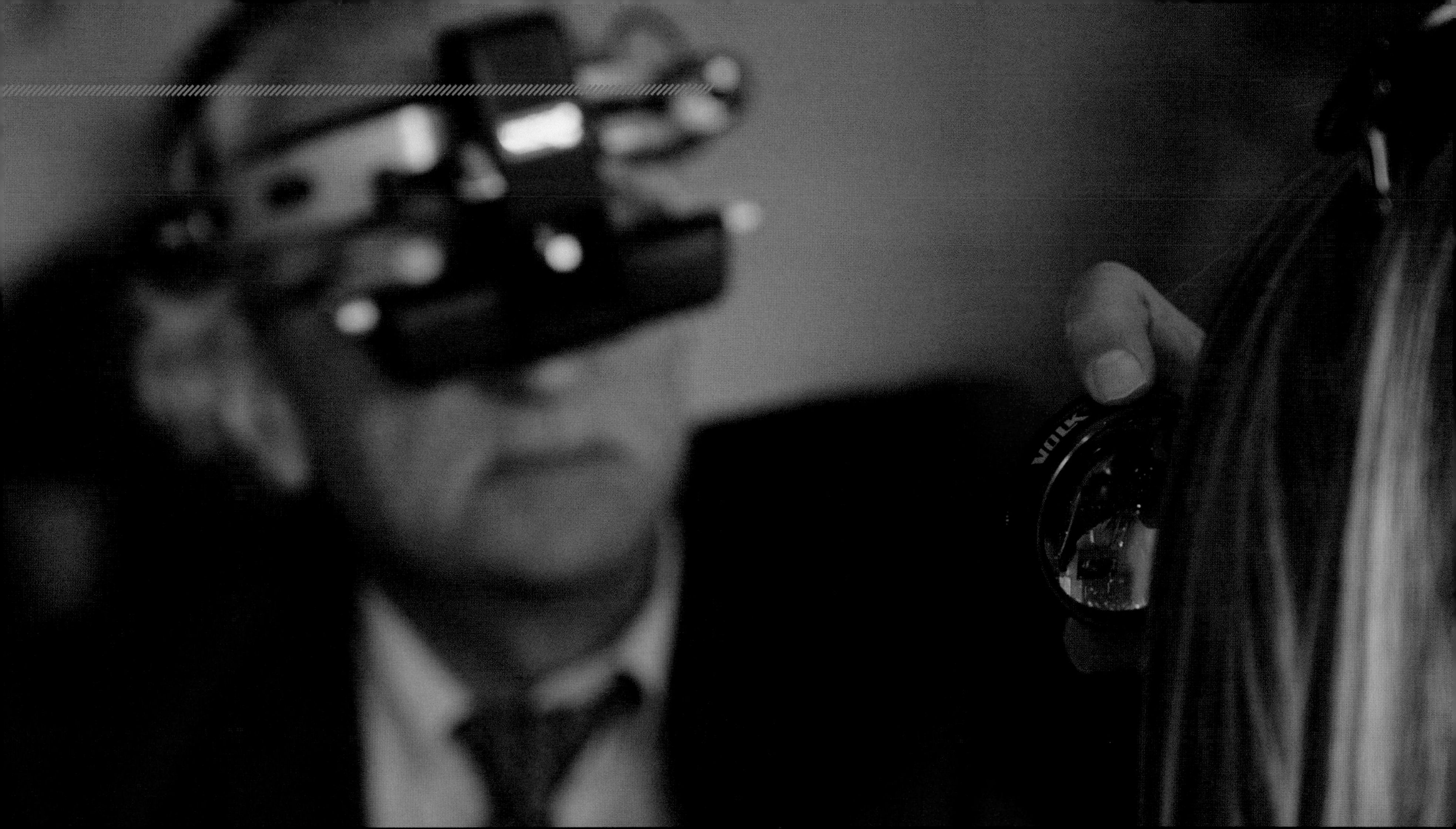
VOLK

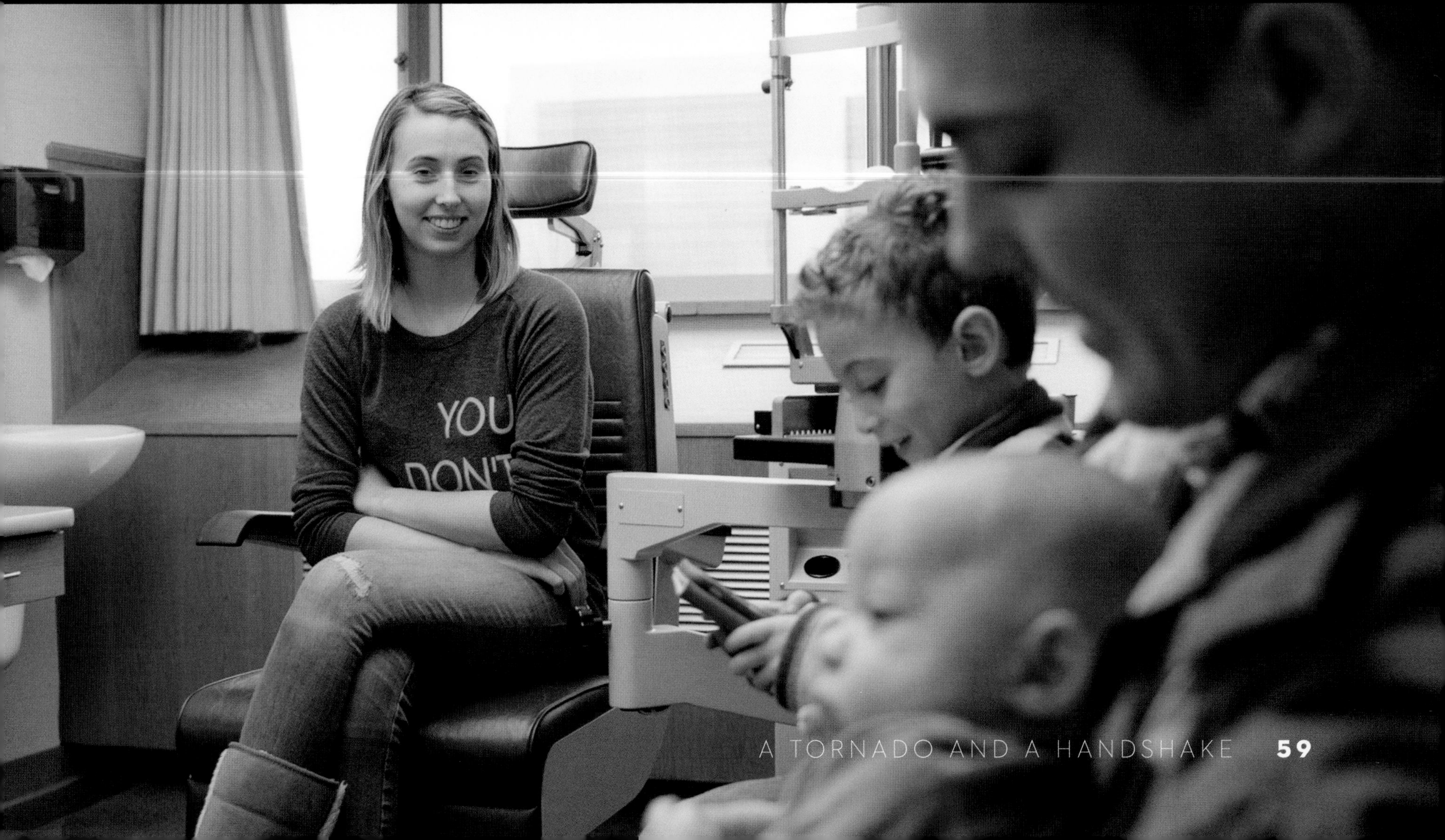
YOU

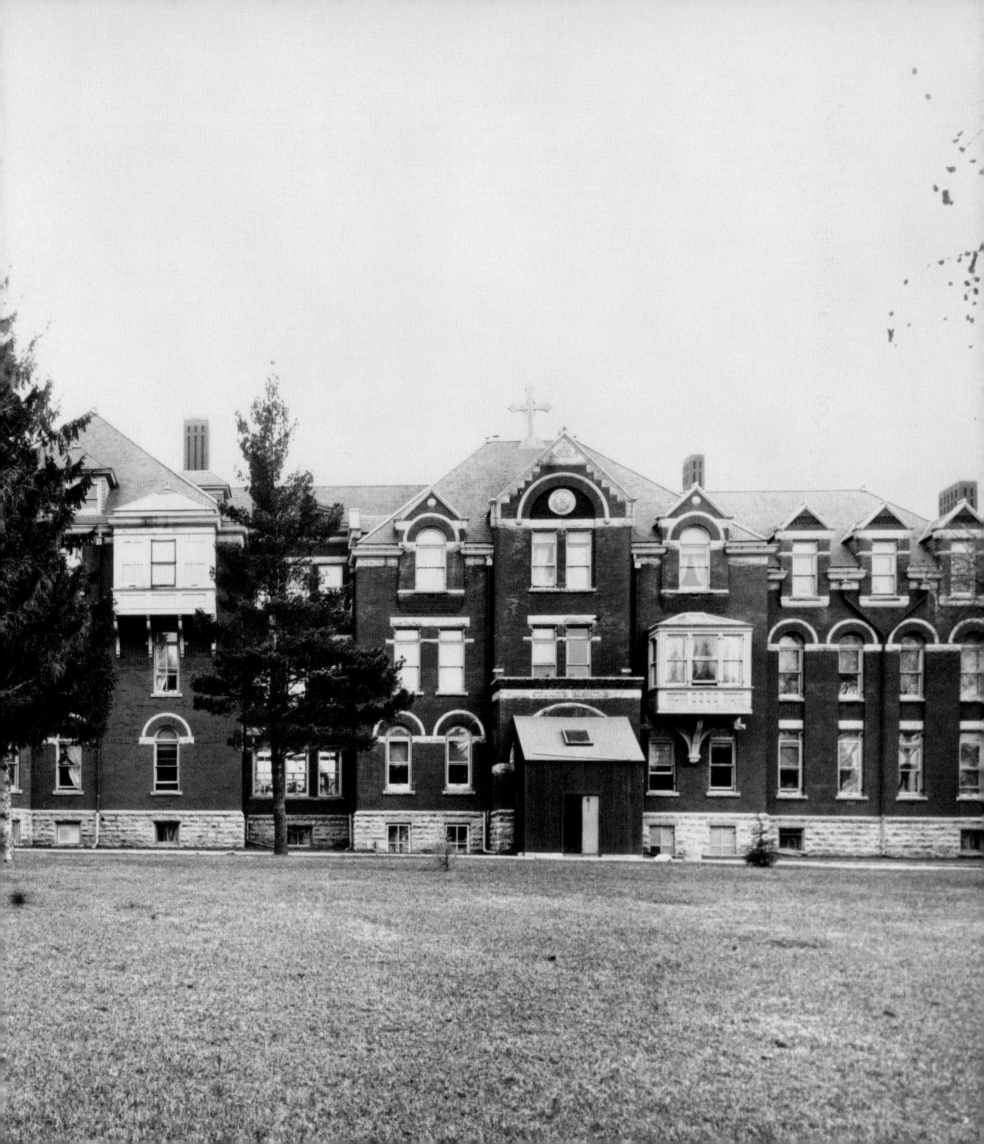

CHAPTER THREE

THE EARLY YEARS

The people will demand, the medical profession must supply, adequate means for the proper care of patients, which means that individualism in medicine can no longer exist.

—DR. WILL MAYO

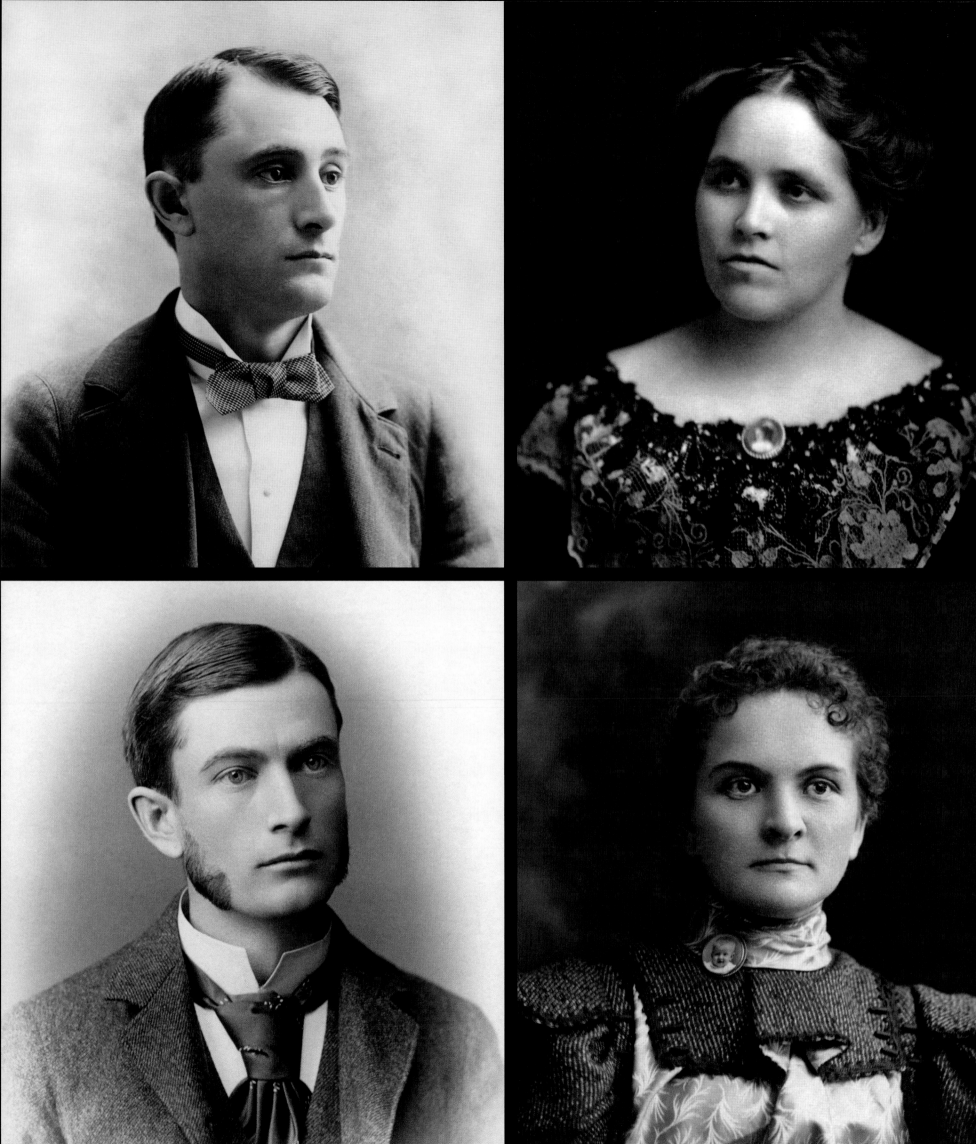

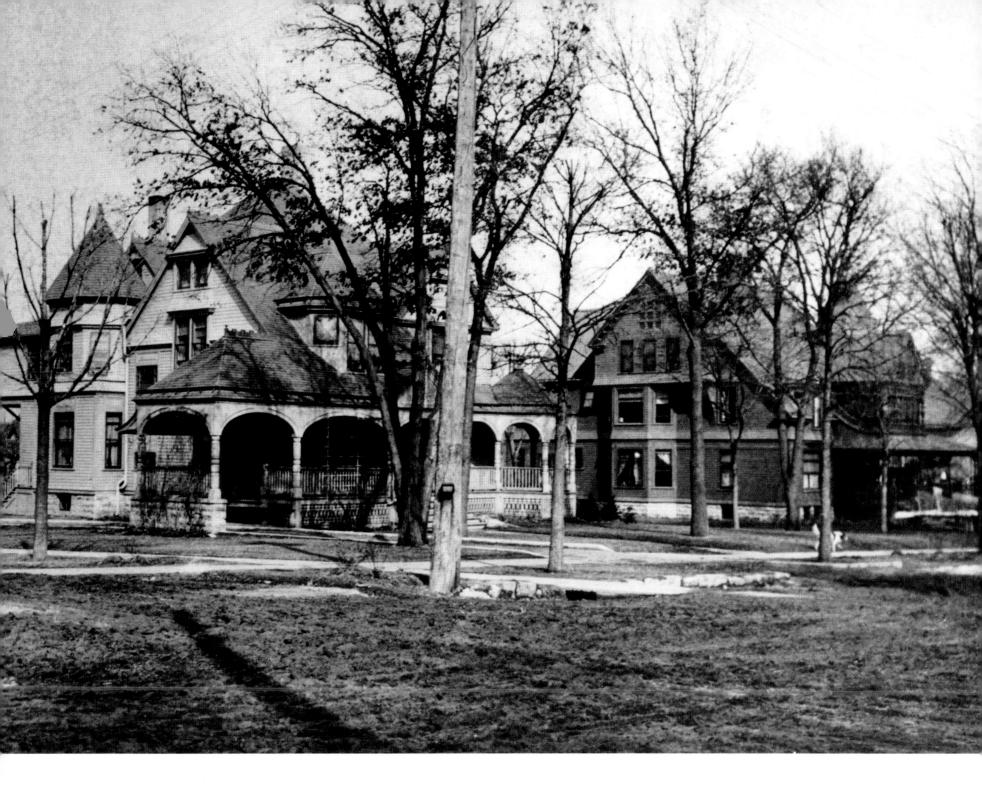

Throughout the 1890s, as Will and Charlie Mayo took over their father's practice, the brothers remained inseparable. They walked to work together. They made decisions together. They built their first homes next to each other. And they shared a bank account, both signing checks simply, "Dr. Mayo."

While they both performed all kinds of surgeries, Charlie specialized in delicate operations on the head and neck. Will, like his father, focused on abdominal and gynecological procedures. Will was authoritative, clear-minded, visionary, a perfectionist. Charlie was more easygoing, less intimidating, friendly. They had their disagreements, but never in public. With them, it was never "I." It was always, "My brother and I."

Will and Charlie, people in town said, were married to the practice. But, like their father, they were also both married to strong women. Will's wife, Hattie, who had grown up in Rochester with the brothers, was shy and formal. An artist, she mostly stayed out of medical affairs, but she designed their houses and served as a hostess to doctors and dignitaries from all over the world. Charlie married Edith Graham, the nurse who instructed the Sisters at Saint Marys. She was the opposite of Hattie—feisty, outgoing, and an integral part of the Mayos' practice.

Opposite, clockwise from top left: *Dr. Charlie, Edith Graham Mayo, Hattie Mayo, Dr. Will*
Above: *the Mayos' homes*

> For someone who is, I would say, nonreligious as Will Mayo was, to refer to the spiritual as being so important for the care of the patients and the good of the clinic to survive, I think just spoke volumes about the Mayo brothers' insights. If we pay too much attention to the material nature of what we do and ignore the spiritual, we will amount to nothing as a clinic.
>
> —ALLEN AKSAMIT JR., M.D.,
> MAYO CLINIC NEUROLOGIST

Sister Joseph Dempsey was the second in a long line of formidable women who would lead Saint Marys Hospital, working closely with the Mayos but also maintaining the Sisters' independence and values. She served as Dr. Will's main surgical assistant for twenty-five years and became so skilled that she would continue with an operation when he turned away to explain something to visiting doctors or students.

Opposite: Sister Joseph Dempsey

The first time Sister Joseph was asked to assist at examining a patient, she ran into a corner of the room and stood facing the wall, outraged and ashamed, because the man was naked. She told Nurse Edith it was impossible for her to be a nurse; she planned to transfer back to teaching immediately. But Edith convinced her to stay, and in less than three years Sister Joseph was head of the hospital.

**—SISTER ELLEN WHELAN , PH.D.,
ORDER OF SAINT FRANCIS, ROCHESTER, MN**

In the late nineteenth, early twentieth century, medicine was highly individualistic. If you were a doctor, you held your skills close to the vest. You were afraid of losing money or prestige or patients.

—MATTHEW DACY, MAYO CLINIC HISTORIAN

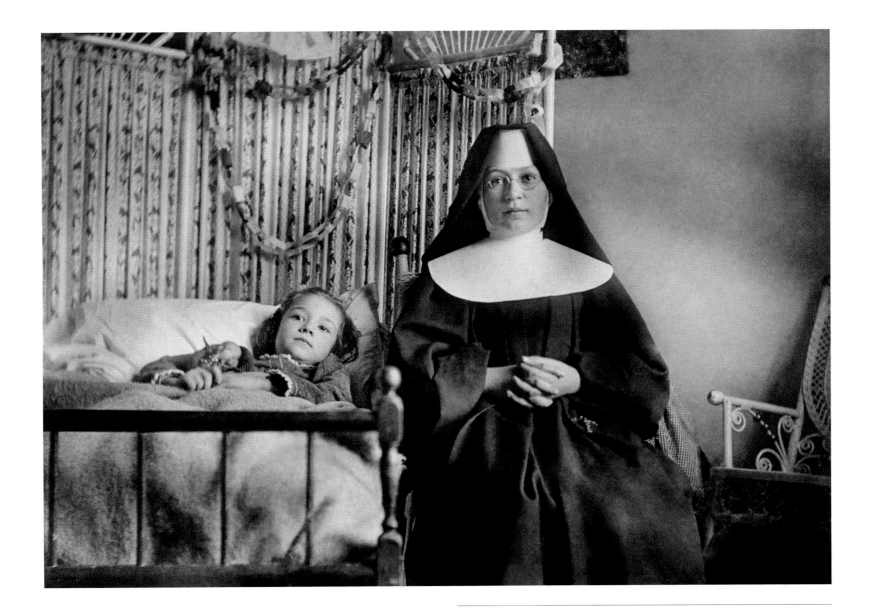

One cold morning, railroad workers in Waterville, Minnesota, removed a window from a passenger car on the Minneapolis–St. Louis Line so they could slide a stretcher in across two seats. On it was 5-year-old Lucy Gray. She was in great pain and had been feverish for almost two weeks. Her parents were taking her to Rochester, Minnesota, where they had heard about some country doctors who were having remarkable success.

A few hours later, Lucy woke up in a dimly lit room at Saint Marys Hospital, recovering from an emergency appendectomy performed by Dr. Charlie. Another hour, and it would have been too late. But an infection set in. There was another operation. And then another. She was not getting better. The Sisters held late-night prayers in their chapel.

The youngest nurse played with Lucy day after day, making a chain of paper rings, each ring representing a day in the hospital, until they decorated the entire screen behind her bed. Lucy Gray lived to age 96. She always gave the Mayo brothers—and the Sisters' faith—equal credit for saving her life.

An autonomous doctor brings to his practice and to the service of his patients the knowledge and experience he has alone. He misses the opportunity to enrich that. When you're talking about health care and people's lives, the value of somebody else's additional knowledge or experience could mean the difference between life and death.

—SISTER TIERNEY TRUEMAN, ORDER OF SAINT FRANCIS, ROCHESTER, MN

Above: Lucy Gray

By 1892, the elder Dr. Mayo was 73 years old. His sons were confidently in charge. He decided to step back from his practice in order to indulge in his other varied interests. He became a Minnesota State Senator, and he loved to travel and tinker with machinery.

To handle the ever-increasing volume of new admissions at Saint Marys, the Mayo brothers began to bring other doctors—including a woman—into their Third Street practice to examine and diagnose patients prior to surgery at the Sisters' hospital. The arrival of these specialists signaled something new and fundamentally transforming—a collaborative approach to medicine.

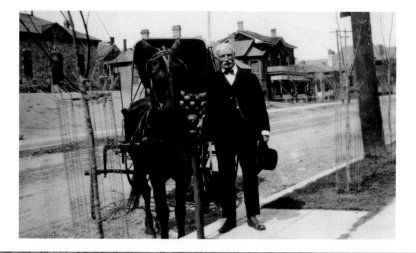

The concept of this multispecialty, teamwork-based group practice for the good of a single patient was maybe the greatest contribution that the Mayo brothers brought to American medicine. When I'm stuck with a patient, and I don't have the answer for a particular patient, I have no hesitation to share that patient with another of my colleagues.

—ALLEN AKSAMIT JR., M.D., MAYO CLINIC NEUROLOGIST

I had a patient with a very unique condition. And within twenty minutes I was able to speak to the various sub-specialties that I needed to contact. In private practice it's really challenging to do that for a lot of different reasons.

—JOHN WALD, M.D., MAYO CLINIC NEURORADIOLOGIST

Teamwork is collective wisdom. Nobody can know everything, and I think that's the beauty of the group practice that the Mayo brothers recognized early on.

—CHRISTOPHER BOES, M.D., MAYO CLINIC NEUROLOGIST

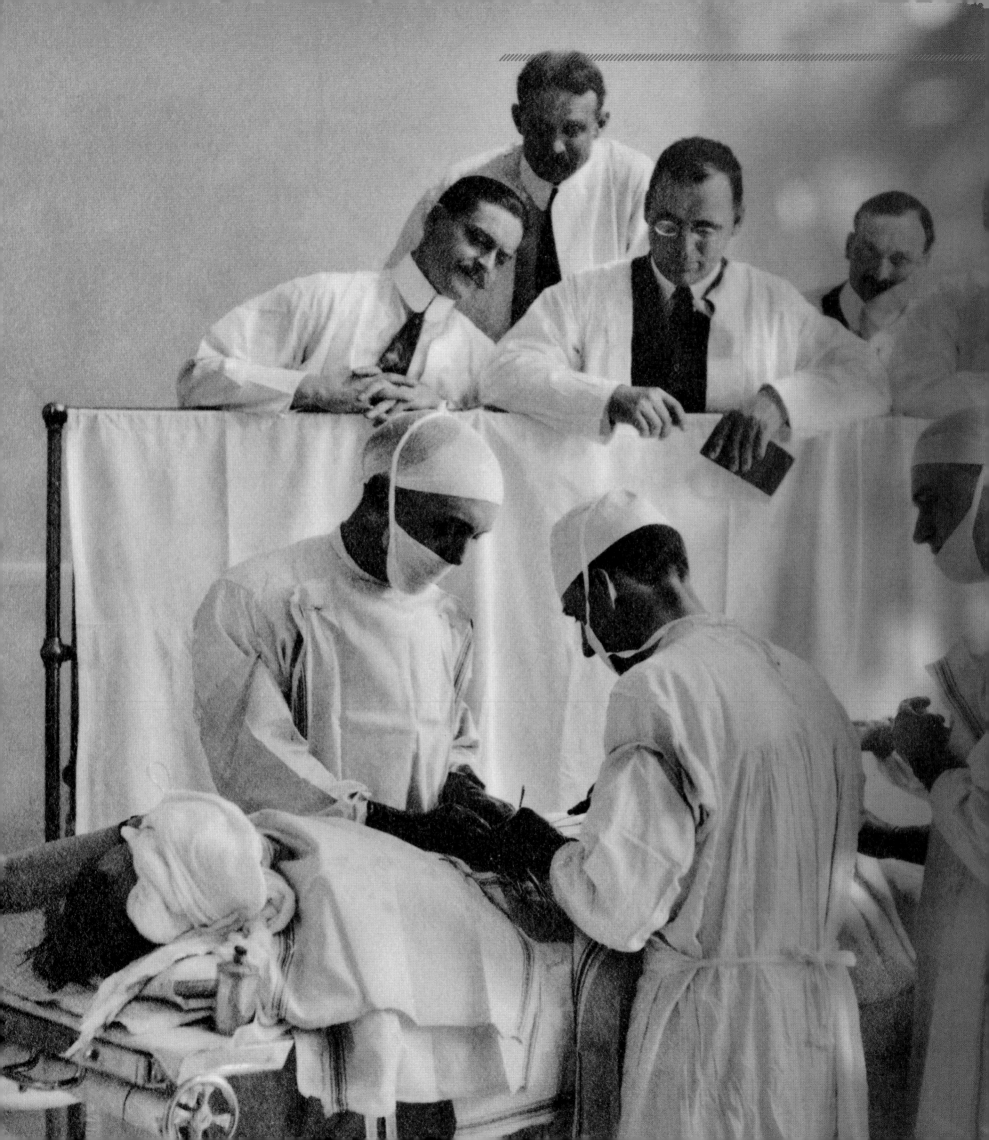

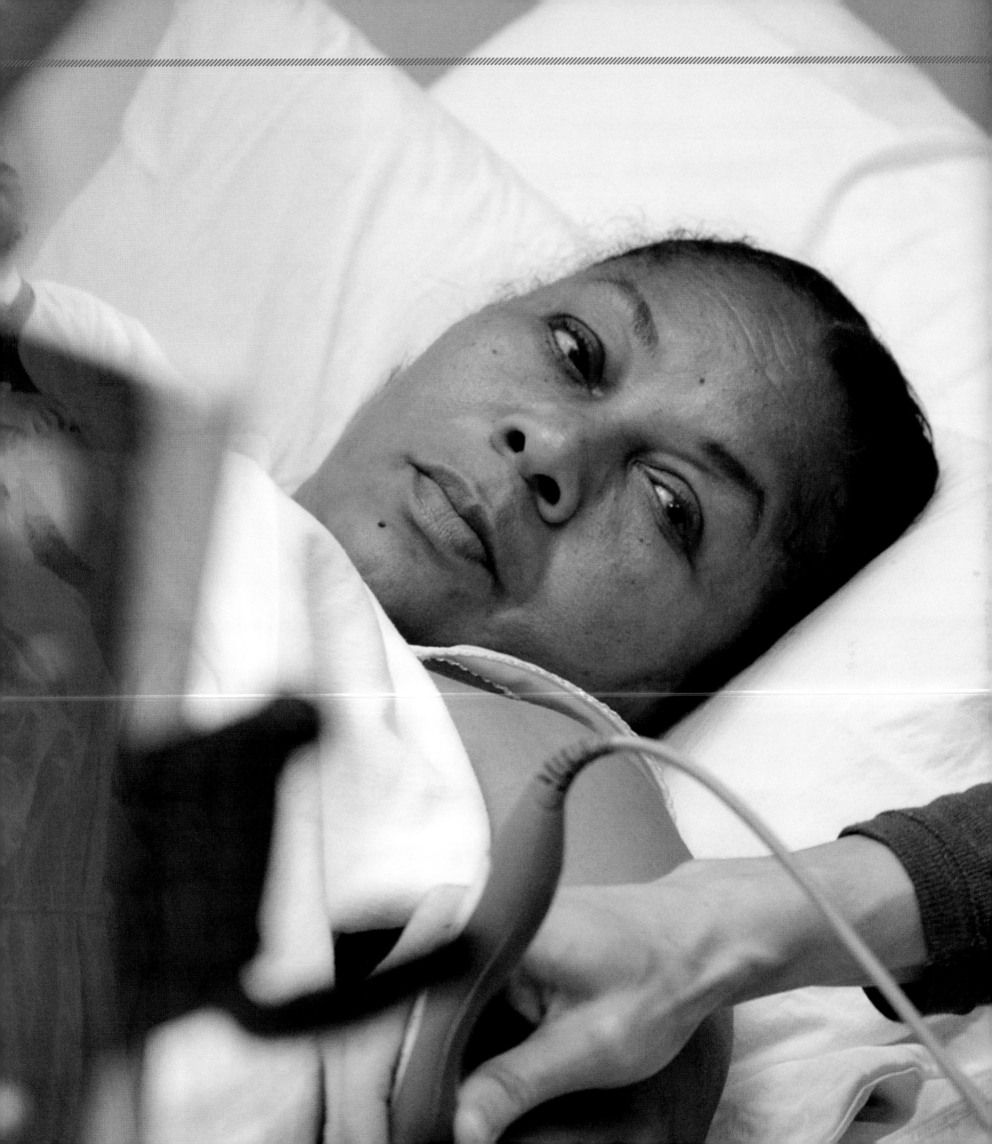

DIAGNOSIS: INCLUSION BODY MYOSITIS, DIABETES, LEUKEMIA

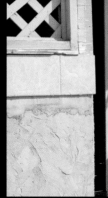
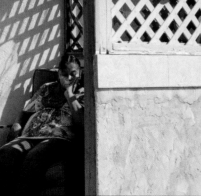

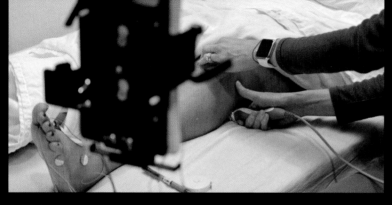

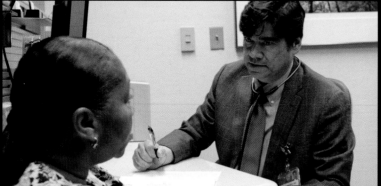

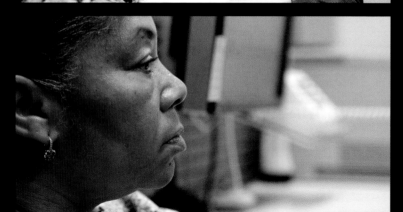

Preamble

CHARLENE KELLY (Jacksonville, FL): All of a sudden your whole world done change on you. When I got up, I couldn't hardly walk. I was shuffling my feet, losing my balance, and I was like, *Wow, there's something going on with me, but what?* I have no idea. The neurologist doctor, he was like, "You have myositis, [and] there's no cure for it." And when you have a doctor who tells you that, it seems like all hope is gone. But I still don't feel like I have the right answer to what's going on with me. Somebody out there may have a different diagnosis. I know people come from around the world to get into Mayo Clinic to get a second opinion. I called in January, but I couldn't get an appointment because they weren't accepting new patients at the time. The young lady told me to call back in December. I didn't mention it to her, but when I got off the phone, I said, "Wow, I hope I be alive," because we're talking about eleven months. During that time while I was waiting, I was going downhill. But I never gave up hope. Never. And so when I got accepted in, that was my world. It is a second opinion on my life. I'm very excited. I'm looking forward to it.

Day 1

CK: Here I am. I don't know if it's gonna be the same diagnosis—that I have myositis—or something else, but I'm hopeful. During the discussion with Dr. Kennelly, she listened to what I was saying. I didn't have that in the past. I mean, she took her time with me, she didn't rush me, she explained everything to me.

KATHLEEN KENNELLY, M.D. (Mayo Clinic neurologist): Inclusion body myositis is a category of muscle disorders that are thought to be inflammatory. It's a tough one because it's kind of creepy-crawly. It doesn't come on like gangbusters: it sneaks up on people.

CK: I noticed they were on the ball of doing different stuff, like checking my blood, that I felt I should have at the early stage, but it wasn't done like that. I come here, and they are on the ball of boom, boom, boom, boom, doing this and that. Thirty minutes later I'm on the road driving home, and Dr. Kennelly called me and said, "I got your test results back." I said, "You got *my* test results back?" Because normally when you take blood, it's a couple of weeks. And she said, "Well, it does look like you have diabetes," and "Have they ever told you that your white cell count is high?"

Day 2

KK: The blood work was important. And her white blood cell count is markedly elevated. For Mrs. Kelly I'm asking for the hematologist to see her and I'm asking for the endocrinology department to see her. I think we will be able to give her a definitive answer. I'm still most suspicious that she has this inclusion body myositis, but it's possible that the elevated white blood cell count could be affecting her

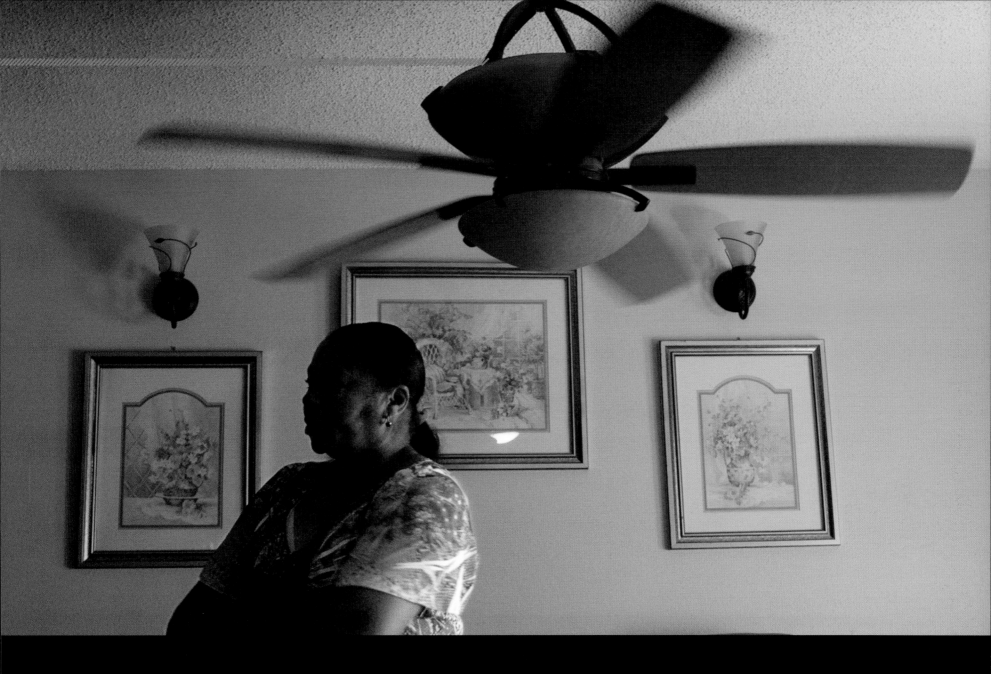

muscles. That has potentially nothing to do with her muscle disease, but it might.

GERARDO COLON-OTERO, M.D. (Mayo Clinic hematologist): They found that her white count is high, which may be an indication of a low-grade leukemia. This is sometimes associated with these muscle inflammatory processes. So we may have the cause.

CK: Leukemia was not something that I thought was going to be told to me. It was devastating.

GC: It's quite likely that she may have had it at least for ten or fifteen years, or even longer. Cranial cell leukemia had been associated with this inclusion body myositis. So we approached her condition with some chemotherapy directed to the leukemia and another medication directed to the myositis.

CK: I went for eight weeks, and I felt like it worked in the beginning. Then my husband lost his job, and I wasn't able to continue to go to the Mayo Clinic because I lost my insurance. I had to seek out other places. What other option do you have? Trying to get in to see someone, it's a battle, you know? Who wants for somebody like me to come in and I've got all these problems? The main thing that comes out of their mouth is, "How would you like to pay for this?" Things cost money. The Mayo Clinic, it's not free. But if I was able to continue the treatments, I felt like the Mayo Clinic was my hope to help me.

GC: I visited with her after she lost her insurance, and was able to examine her and determine where we stood with her treatment. Her condition doesn't seem to have improved that much.

CK: You know, sometimes it doesn't work like you want it to in the beginning. I got weaker. But he looked me dead in my eye and said, "You're gonna live a long life. You can live a long life with leukemia. All hope is not gone." They did all they could do for me. I thank them from the bottom of my heart for giving me answers to what I was looking for. You know you just have to move on, and that's what I'm trying to do now. I knew in the beginning it was gonna be a journey, and it still is a journey—and it's still going.

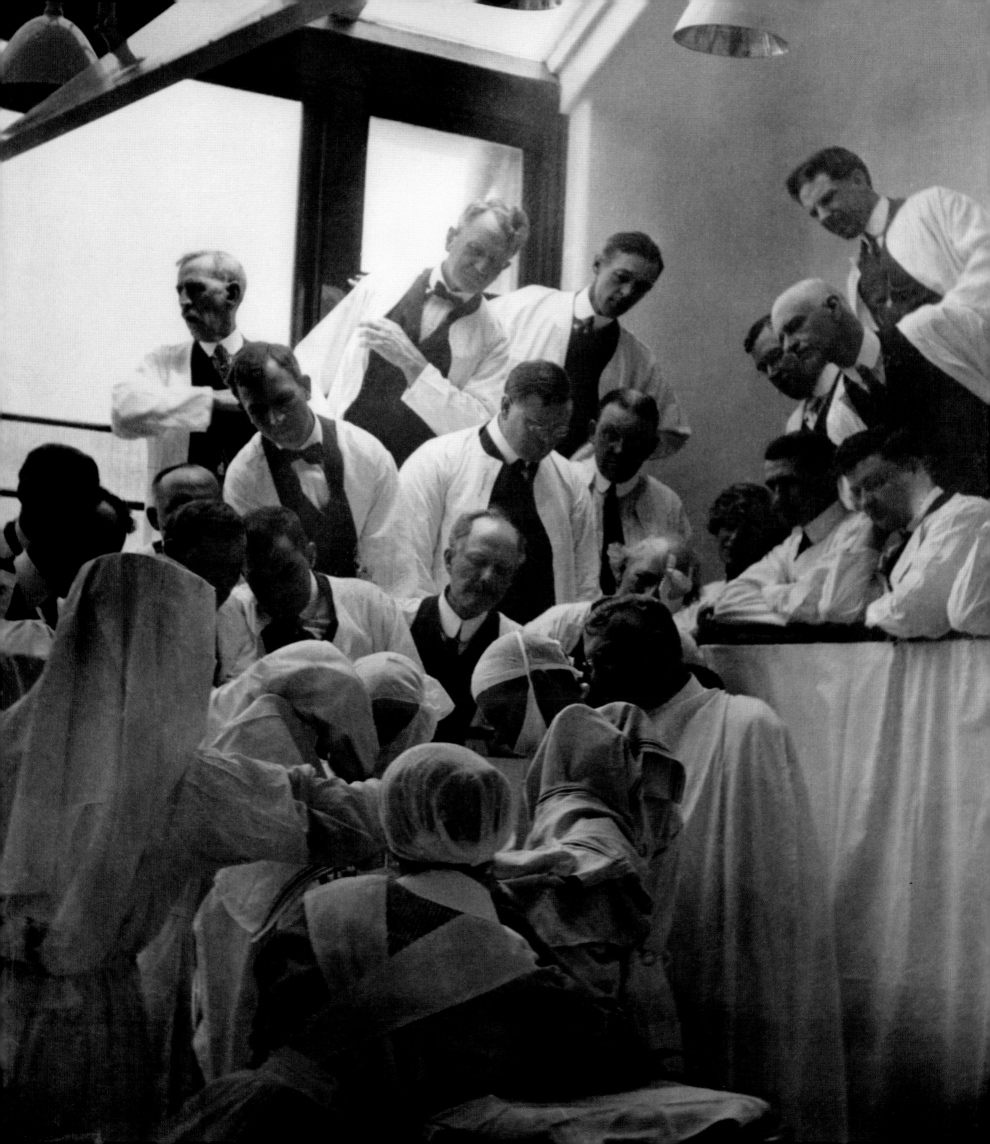

THE NEEDS
OF THE PATIENT
COME FIRST

Their hospital in the little prairie city of not more than 5,000 inhabitants has become a Mecca for surgeons....There is no other hospital on this side of the Atlantic in which so many important operations are performed daily.

—NICHOLAS SENN, M.D.

As the twentieth century dawned, there was not yet a formal medical center in Rochester, Minnesota. There was simply a small but unique group practice, now on the second floor of the Masonic Building, led by two surgeons and several associates, affiliated with a hospital a mile down the road that was run by a small community of nuns.

After watching the Mayos operate, a well-known Chicago physician reported to his colleagues that the brothers were far more advanced than most surgeons. Patients had been spreading the word about the Mayo brothers for years. Now, more doctors began to travel to Rochester to observe, learn, and even be treated themselves. Eventually, Charlie had to design a custom platform alongside the operating table, with slanting mirrors above it, to accommodate the ever-increasing number of surgeons who just wanted to see them work.

Both men were entirely frank about their role, constantly telling visitors where they had picked up this good thing or that…Dr. Will would say, "I used to do this differently, but Moynihan showed me his method when he was here and it was better, so I use it now." …And Dr. Charlie: "The first time I tried this operation I got stuck at this point, but Dr. George Monk of Boston was here and he told me what to do."

—HELEN CLAPESATTLE, AUTHOR

The Mayo brothers really developed their own continuing medical education program. If they heard about a new procedure, they would go and see that physician, watch him do the new surgery, learn the ins and outs of it, and come back and apply it to Mayo. They took what others did, applied it to a very large number of patients, and really kind of perfected it. And that still goes on.

—CHRISTOPHER BOES, M.D., MAYO CLINIC NEUROLOGIST

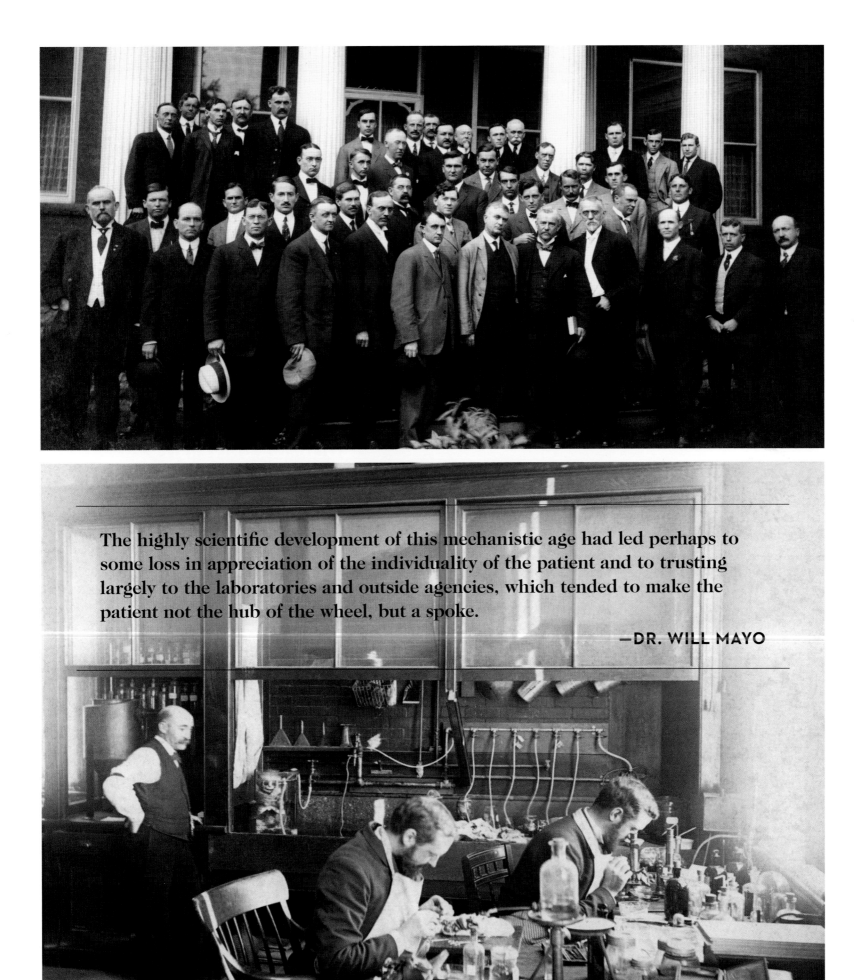

The highly scientific development of this mechanistic age had led perhaps to some loss in appreciation of the individuality of the patient and to trusting largely to the laboratories and outside agencies, which tended to make the patient not the hub of the wheel, but a spoke.

—DR. WILL MAYO

One of the things the Mayos did very successfully around the early 1900s was that the patient became the center, and the doctors orbited around the patient. They refocused the circle of care.

—SIDDHARTHA MUKHERJEE, M.D., PH.D., ONCOLOGIST, AUTHOR, COLUMBIA UNIVERSITY

On most nights, visiting doctors gathered at the "Surgeons Club," where they discussed what they had seen that day. Increasingly, they began to refer to the place where they had witnessed the brothers' extraordinary work as "The Mayos' Clinic at Saint Marys."

Each year, one brother would take an extended educational "vacation" to study different surgical techniques, while the other remained at the practice. Dr. Charlie and his wife, Edith, even attended surgeries during their honeymoon. And, by the 1920s, Dr. Will had witnessed procedures by surgeons in every town in America and Canada with a population of more than 100,000, and had crossed the Atlantic thirty times.

In 1901, the Mayo brothers hired a young doctor, Henry Plummer, who had impressed them with his knowledge of blood diseases. They wanted to focus on surgery, but Plummer helped convince them that better, more advanced lab and diagnostic work would improve surgical outcomes—or perhaps make those surgeries unnecessary. Plummer immediately began modernizing the Mayos' labs and exploring ways to make all the patient information they were gathering more accessible.

William Worrall Mayo had kept long narratives about patients on the back of ledger pages. Later, his sons and the doctors who joined the practice kept their own separate individual case notes. Henry Plummer was determined to standardize their records.

Each physician would record the patient's information, but then when the patient came back, they might not have seen the same physician, and so they didn't know what the other physician had told the patient. And so it was very difficult to know how to treat or move forward with treatment.

—RENEE ZIEMER, MAYO CLINIC HISTORIAN

Opposite, top left: Henry Plummer

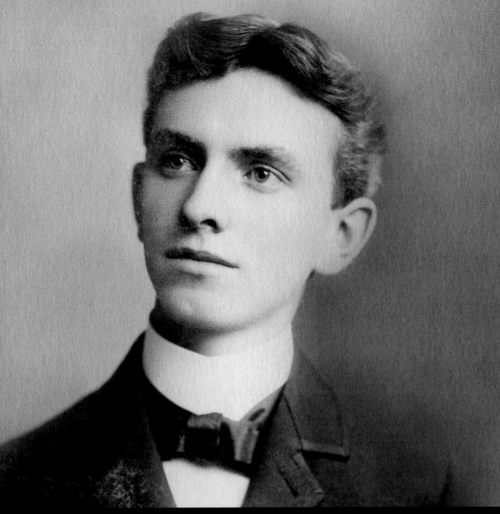

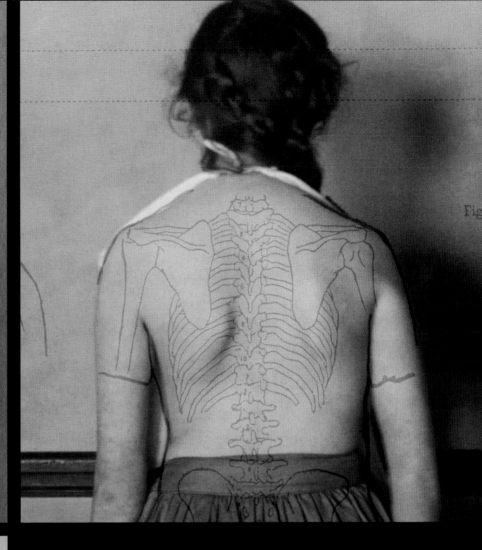

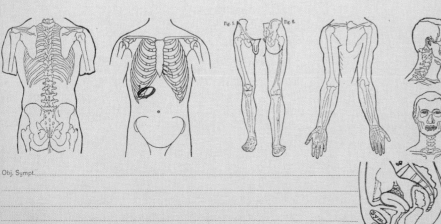

The genius of Plummer's invention was to say, the heart does not live in the cardiologist's office, the lung doesn't live in the pulmonologist's office, the spine doesn't live in the orthopedist's office. They're part of the same person. To reflect that wholeness, you need to have a medical record that is attached not to the doctor's offices but to the patient individually, and not just in one single moment of time, but through all time. Plummer's invention eventually spread throughout the whole nation—actually through the world.

—SIDDHARTHA MUKHERJEE, M.D., PH.D.

> On a bitter day in January 1905, Dr. Wilson put the pathology specimen on the windowsill, froze it, and with a little bit of colored dye could assess in one stop whether the patient had cancer.
>
> —MATTHEW DACY, MAYO CLINIC HISTORIAN

On July 1, 1907, a 48-year-old housewife from British Columbia arrived in Rochester with intense nerve pain, fever, and chills. The diagnosis was a gallbladder infection. After a successful surgery, she went home. For Henry Plummer and his new system, she was Patient Number 1.

The Mayo brothers also hired a pathologist named Louis Wilson. Dr. Will challenged him to develop a reliable way to tell if a tissue was cancerous while the patient was still on the operating table. At the time, preparing tissue samples for analysis took days. Wilson developed an ingenious way to get specimens under the microscope in less than two minutes.

Dr. Wilson now insisted that his lab be situated next to the operating room, a practice that continues to this day.

> Literally in a matter of minutes, he could go back and tell the operating surgeon, "It's not a malignant tumor," or, "The margins of the edges of the tumor you've taken out don't show any tumor; you don't have to operate further."
>
> —BRUCE FYE, M.D.,
> MAYO CLINIC MEDICAL HISTORIAN

Just a few feet from where we are right now, there's a massive pathology lab with multiple technicians in there freezing, cutting, and staining slides, and two pathologists reading it. There's nothing like that anywhere in the world. The speed with which we get people answers is great. I know by the time I talk to the family after the operation if the margins are clear. It's a great burden lifted off them to hear that immediately.

—RORY SMOOT, M.D., MAYO CLINIC GENERAL SURGEON

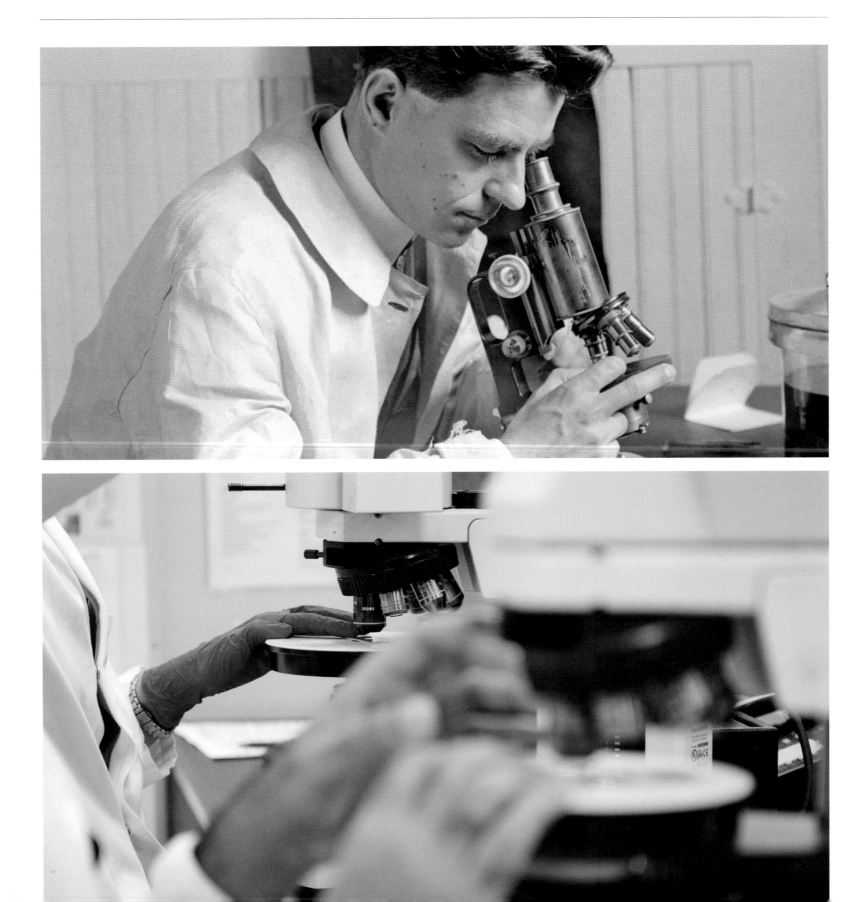

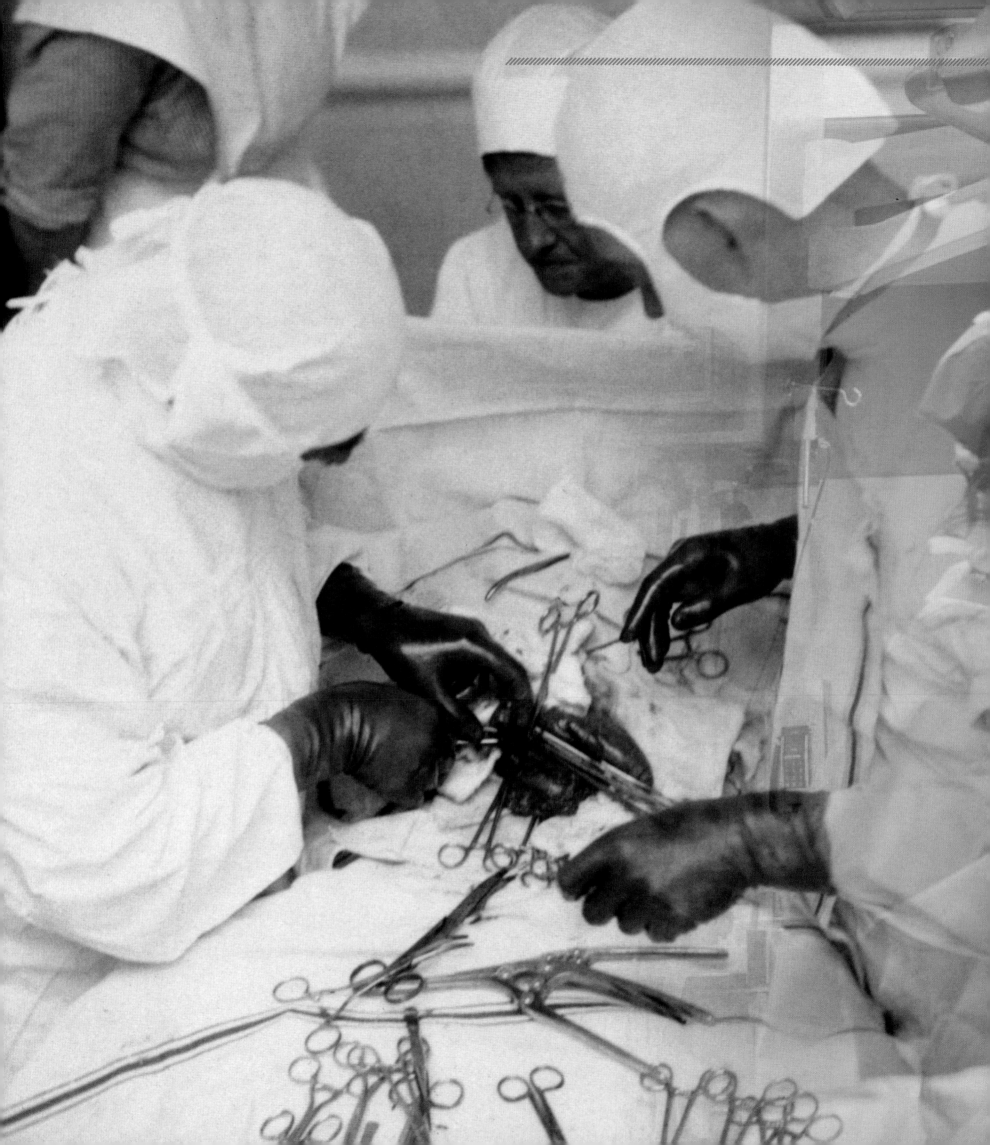

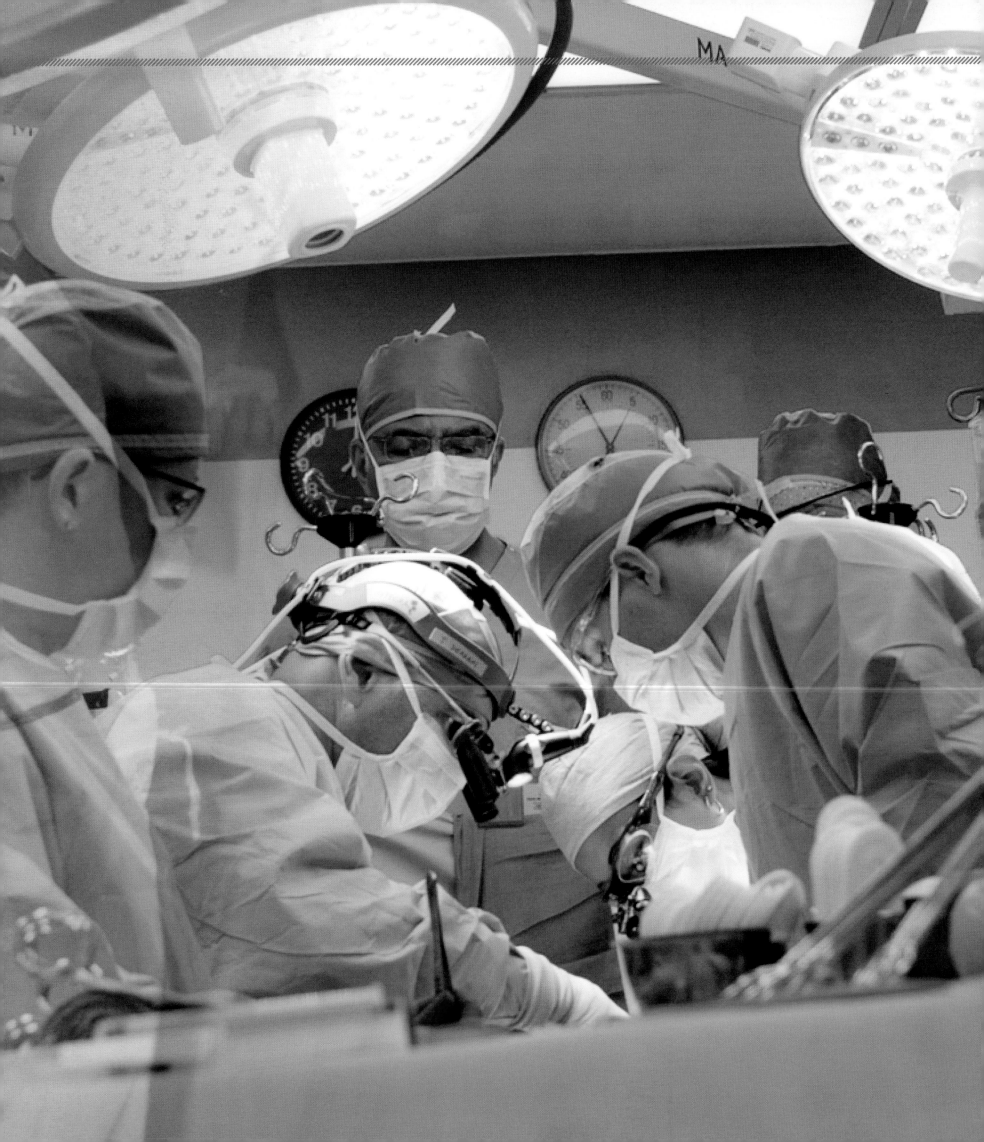

ANNA JENKINS (Durham, NC): I was diagnosed with Ebstein's anomaly when I was born. It's a disease of the heart. In my case, half the blood is sent in the wrong direction. And that causes the heart not to function as efficiently. I've had the same cardiologist almost my whole life. The only reason we decided not to stay in North Carolina for this surgery was because of Dr. Dearani's experience. The surgeon at home has only done fifteen Ebstein's anomaly surgeries. But Dr. Dearani has managed to do 800. So the sheer numbers were just unbelievable.

JOSEPH DEARANI, M.D. (Mayo Clinic cardiac surgeon): We are a destination medical center, which means there are many patients who will travel for answers. With Anna, it was a surgeon who referred her to me—one of my colleagues; a very, very good surgeon. With Anna's case, she's an elite athlete, and the heart is getting progressively enlarged.

AJ: The analogy Dr. Dearani gave me was a spring. If you stretch a spring—which is what happens with athletics—it'll bounce back. But if you stretch a spring way too far, it gets stuck. And that's what we don't want to happen. I'm a little nervous. Although I don't think I'm as nervous as my parents are. It would have been convenient to stay at home and not to have flights and be living out of a hotel room for a week. And I know the recovery will be long, but if my heart enlarges any more, I will not be able to do any of the athletics I do. I may not even be able to walk up the stairs anymore.

AJ (post-op): My nurse just brought me a rock. It's shaped like a heart. She said she brought it to bring me peace. And once my chest plate heals, in six to eight weeks down the road, I hope to get back into rowing and join the team and not be too far behind. I think my heart is in a good place.

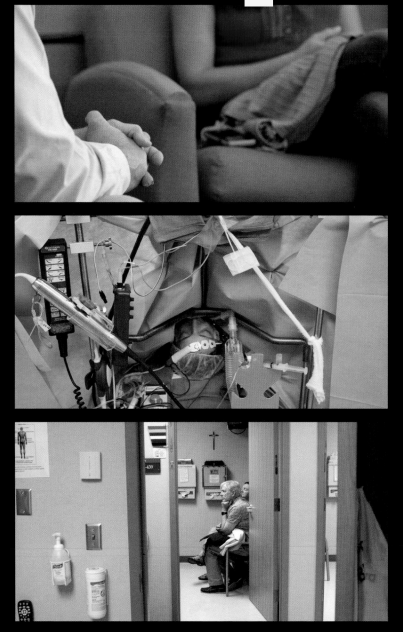

From a patient standpoint, it means that they come in, they can undergo one operation to have their tumor removed, and they can move past that day and start getting on with their lives. Most institutions don't have the support of their pathology department. A woman goes to the operating room to remove a one- or two-centimeter cancer, and then the pathology report may come back a week or two weeks after surgery, and the doctor says, "Well, the margin is positive, so we need to consider a second operation." Sometimes they have to do a third operation.

—JUDY BOUGHEY, M.D., MAYO CLINIC BREAST SURGICAL ONCOLOGIST

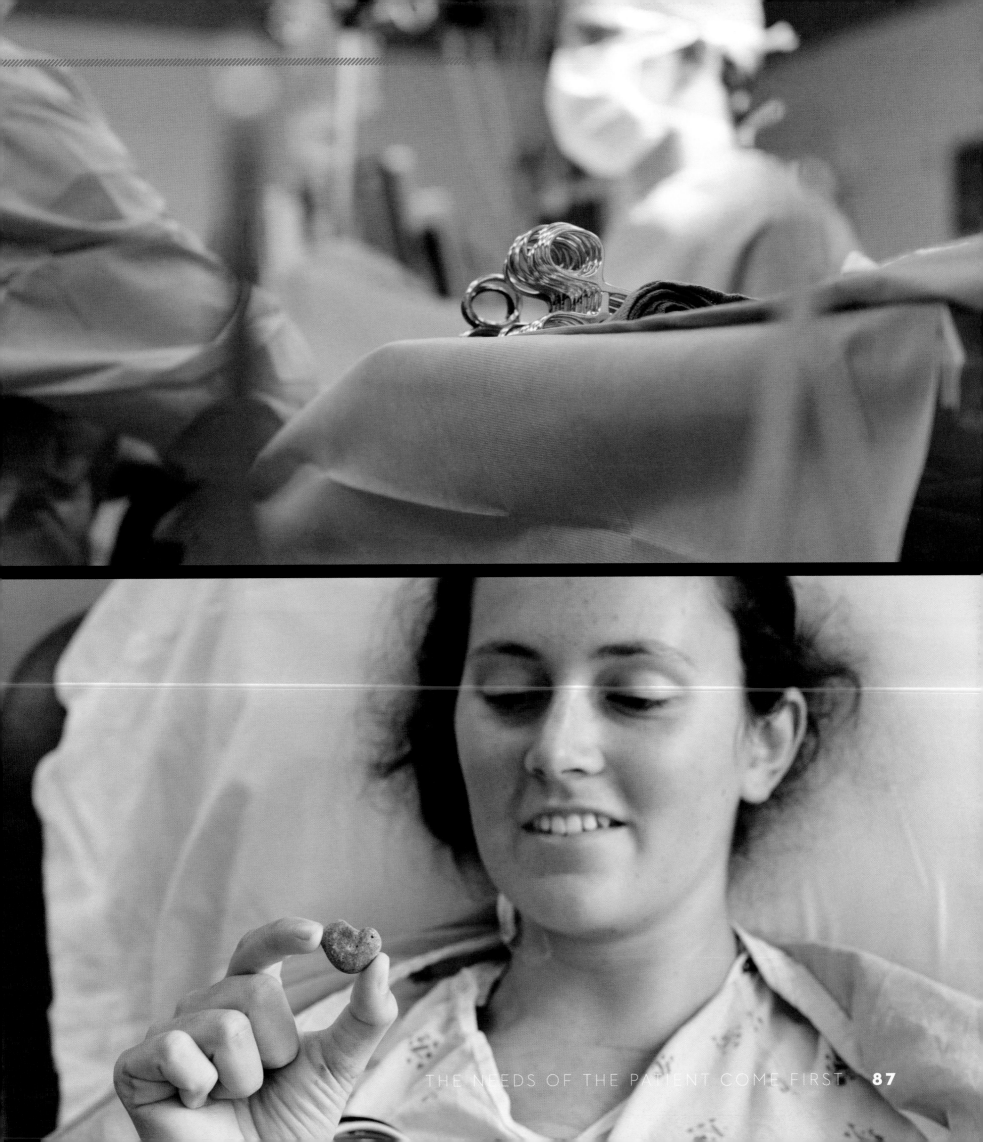

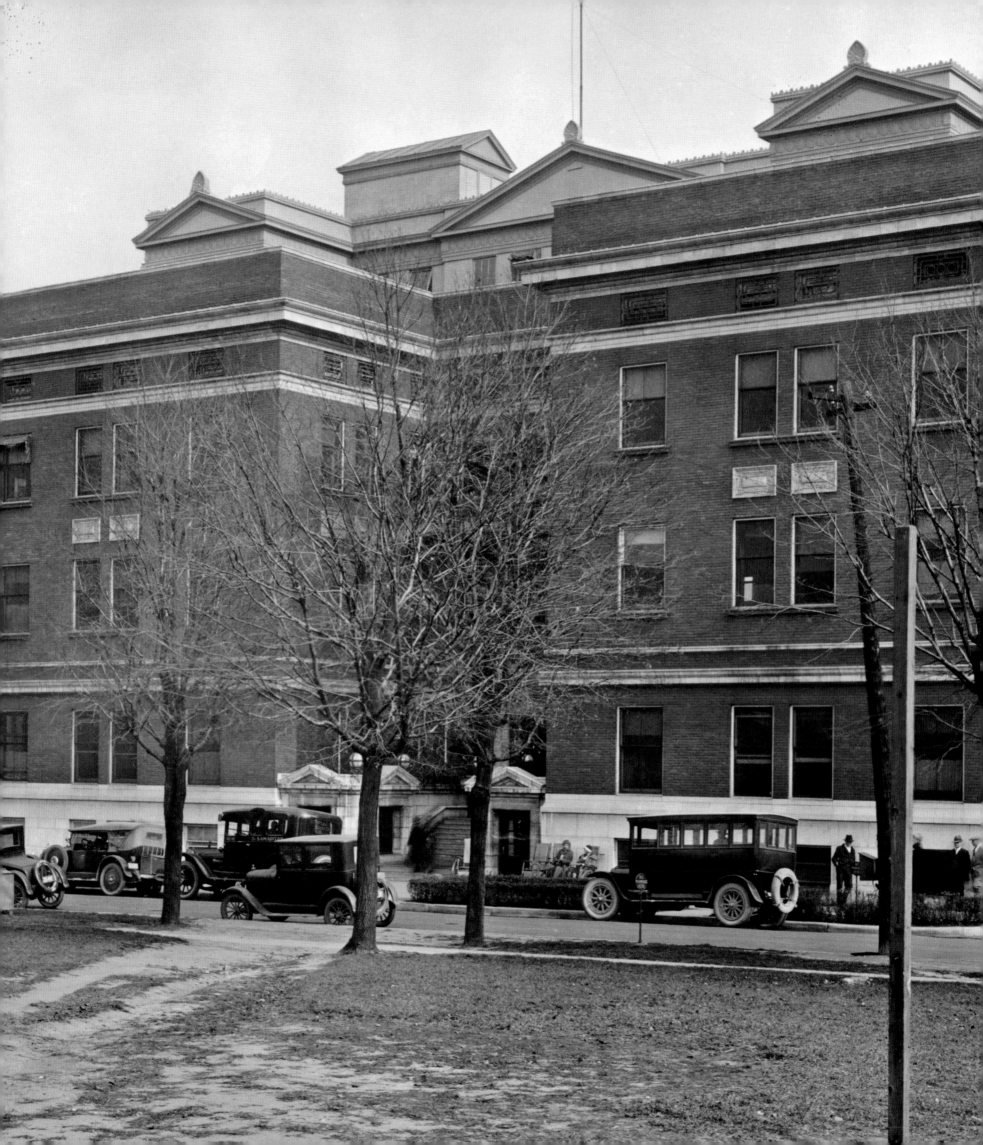

PATIENT CARE, RESEARCH, AND EDUCATION

The gracious privilege is not often accorded mortal man to live to witness the accomplishment, the culmination of his best wishes, his ideals. That this happiness had come to me after many days fills my heart with deepest gratitude and peace.

—WILLIAM WORRALL MAYO, M.D.

In 1905, there were more operations performed at Saint Marys Hospital than at Johns Hopkins. And that's when Rochester had a population of 7,000 and Baltimore had a population of half a million.

—BRUCE FYE, M.D., MAYO CLINIC MEDICAL HISTORIAN

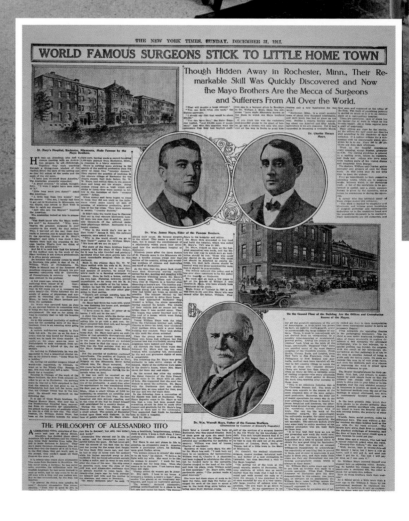

The almost mystical reputation of the Mayo brothers meant more patients. More patients meant more diagnoses. More diagnoses meant more surgeries. More surgeries meant more nurses. And all of it meant more hospital rooms.

There had already been three additions to Saint Marys. What began in 1889 as a small community hospital with only a dozen iron cots ready for patients was now one of the largest and most advanced surgical centers in the United States, where more than 3,000 operations were performed each year. Patients kept coming—from all over the world.

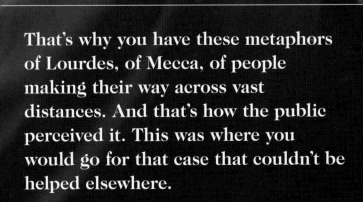

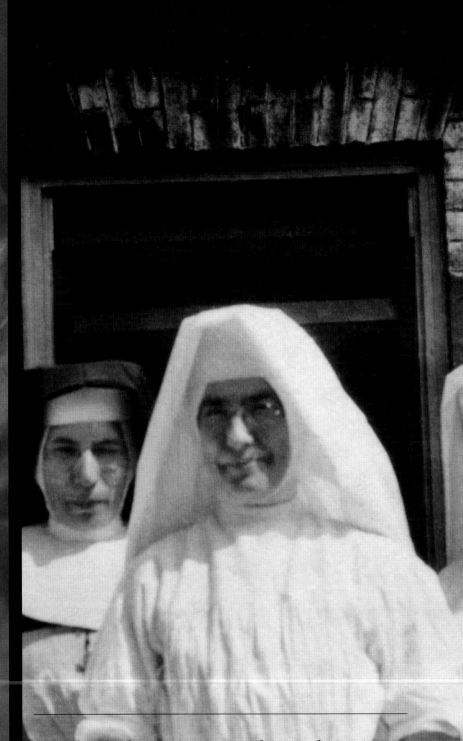

That's why you have these metaphors of Lourdes, of Mecca, of people making their way across vast distances. And that's how the public perceived it. This was where you would go for that case that couldn't be helped elsewhere.

—MATTHEW DACY,
MAYO CLINIC HISTORIAN

I think there are many things that really qualified the Sisters to be nurses. I think it was their empathetic approach to patient care, the humility they brought to their work, and how they worked with each other. It was their Franciscan values, which we really carry into the work that we do today.

—PAMELA JOHNSON, R.N., CHIEF
NURSING OFFICER, MAYO CLINIC

On November 19, 1906, Saint Marys Hospital Training School for Nurses opened its doors. The curriculum combined lectures on anatomy, physiology, and bacteriology, along with classes in practical nursing and hygiene. Students were required to attend at least eight autopsies.

Evidence of the Sisters' faith—and the Mayos' generosity—was everywhere. When Dr. Will learned that a farmer had mortgaged his farm to pay for his surgery, he not only returned the check, but also sent some extra money to help the family until the man recovered.

Nursing is definitely the front line of medicine. We are with the patients 24/7. We are monitoring them 24/7. And we are going to be the first to try and make things better. I know that the Sisters started it, and I think there's a sense of pride in that. There would be many nights when I'd be leaving work at 8, 9 o'clock at night, and Sister Generose would be rolling up her sleeves. I remember Sister Vera, walking the halls when she was 101 or 102, something like that. Let's face it: We can't compete with the Sisters, but if we could do a little fraction of what they've been able to do, it would be an honor. I would like to think that tradition can carry on.

—KATE WELP, R.N., MAYO CLINIC CARDIAC SURGERY CARE UNIT

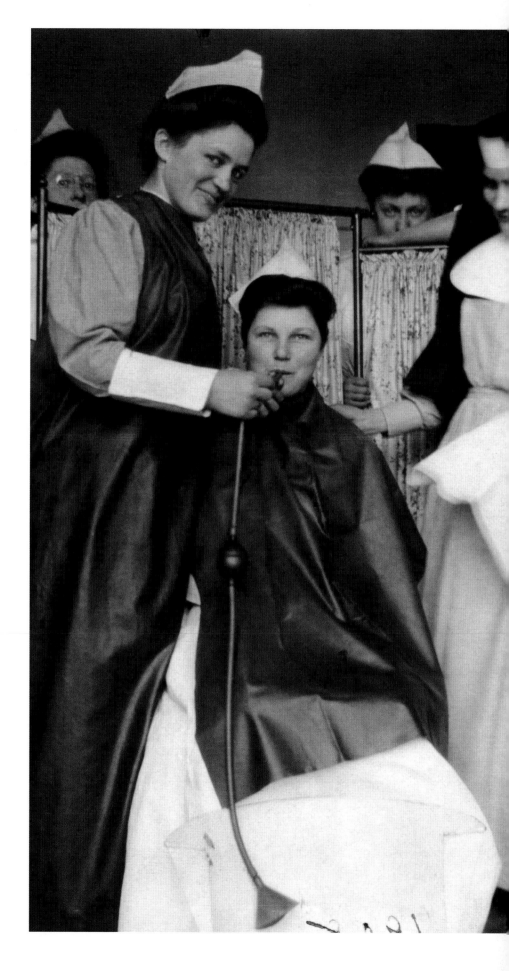

Sister Cashell—one of the nuns here who I sat down with—said that when she went through the nursing school, everyone was taught to look at every patient like Jesus Christ.

—KENDALL LEE, M.D., PH.D., MAYO CLINIC NEUROSURGEON

In small towns the populace really had very little money—often, almost no money. As the Mayo practice grew and more well-to-do patients traveled to Rochester, they would see how much an individual was capable of paying and charge accordingly. The individual, if they were well-to-do, should be able to recognize that. On the other hand, for poorer patients who didn't have the means, they used the sort of principle of Robin Hood: They took the fees they got from the wealthy individuals and they spread those over to cover the cost of care for the poor.

—BRUCE FYE, M.D., MAYO CLINIC MEDICAL HISTORIAN

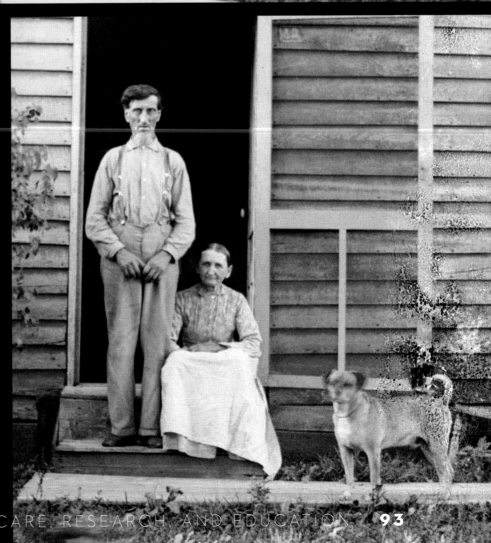

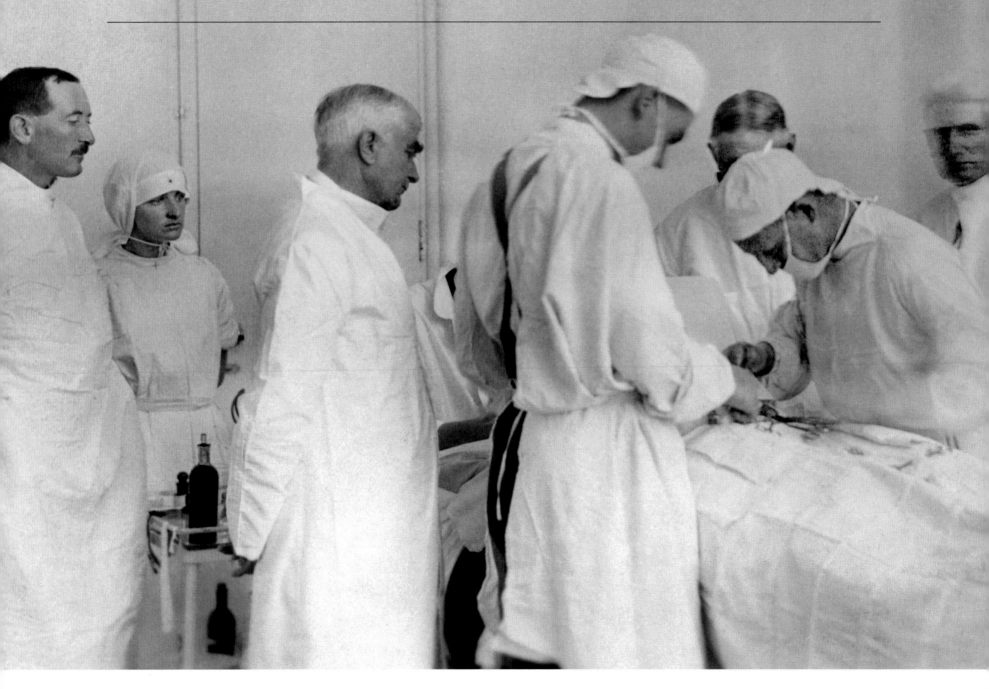

My interest and my brother's interest is to train men for the service of humanity. What can I do with one pair of hands? But, if I can train fifty or five hundred pairs of hands, I have ... [implanted] ideals and scientific spirit in many who in endless chains will carry on the same endeavor.

—DR. WILL MAYO

All along, the brothers maintained their exhaustive schedules. One visiting doctor claimed to have seen Dr. Charlie remove a cataract, tonsils, and a goiter; resect ribs after draining fluid from a patient's lung; perform a complex surgery to reconnect the stomach and intestines; treat a uterine abnormality; correct bowlegs; and cut off bunions—all before going home for lunch.

In 1910, while trying to fix a machine he had constructed to make ethanol from corn, W.W.'s hand was crushed. His son Charlie had to amputate. There were complications. Infections set in. His sons couldn't save him. Dr. William Worrall Mayo, the doctor whose unorthodox collaboration with the Sisters of Saint Francis had transformed the practice of medicine, died on March 6, 1911. He was 91 years old.

By the time W.W. died, it was clear that the Mayo brothers' practice had outgrown its space in the Masonic Temple, as well as the temporary offices they had been renting around town. They needed their own building.

The five-story structure, designed by Henry Plummer, opened on March 6, 1914. It stood on the site of W.W. and Louise's first home, where Dr. Charlie had been born 50 years earlier. Etched in stone over the front entrance were the two words that people had been using for years: "Mayo Clinic."

In addition to dozens of rooms for examinations, diagnostic procedures, and outpatient surgeries, there were clinical and research laboratories, a library, an assembly hall, a pathology museum, and an artist's studio to illustrate illnesses. The medical records department alone took up fifteen rooms.

In February 1915, the Mayo brothers endowed the Mayo Foundation for Medical Education and Research with the University of Minnesota. Their goal was to set a higher standard for training medical specialists. It ultimately made Mayo one of the largest centers of graduate medical education in the world.

The brothers grew up in the Gilded Age, and vast fortunes were being made. But they had grown up seeing their father waive or reduce his charges, and they were inspired by the Franciscan Sisters. Dr. Will and Charlie believed that if you have certain skills, abilities, and resources, you hold them in trust to give back to other people. And they applied that through the profession of medicine.

—MATTHEW DACY, MAYO CLINIC HISTORIAN

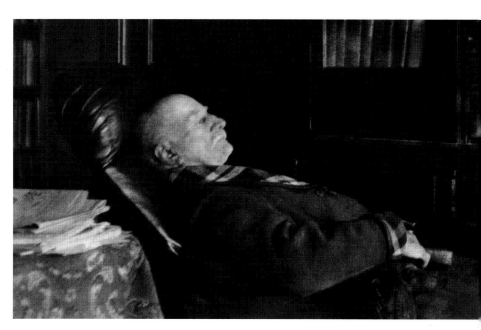

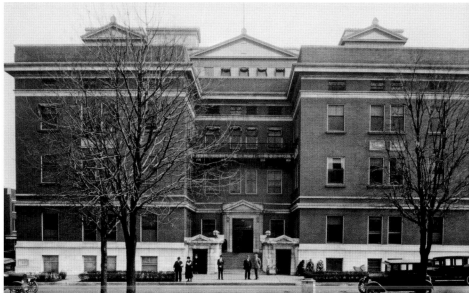

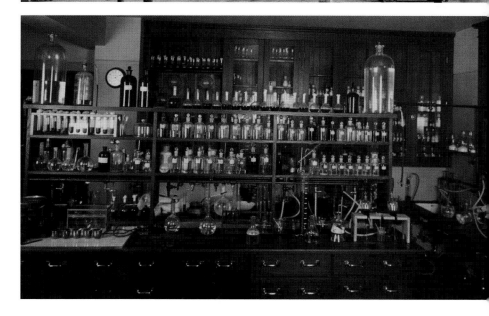

Education is core to Mayo's being. Will and Charlie invested heavily in it. It's the premise on which the future of Mayo will lie, because we're trying to embody that level of teamwork and all that we do for every young person who decides to get an education here. They see the future and see something that they can build that's greater than what they've inherited.

**—EDDIE GREENE, M.D.,
MAYO CLINIC NEPHROLOGIST**

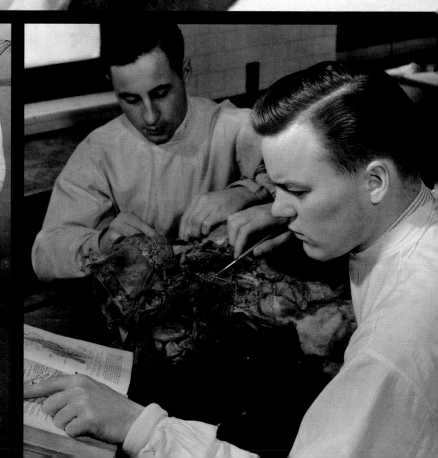

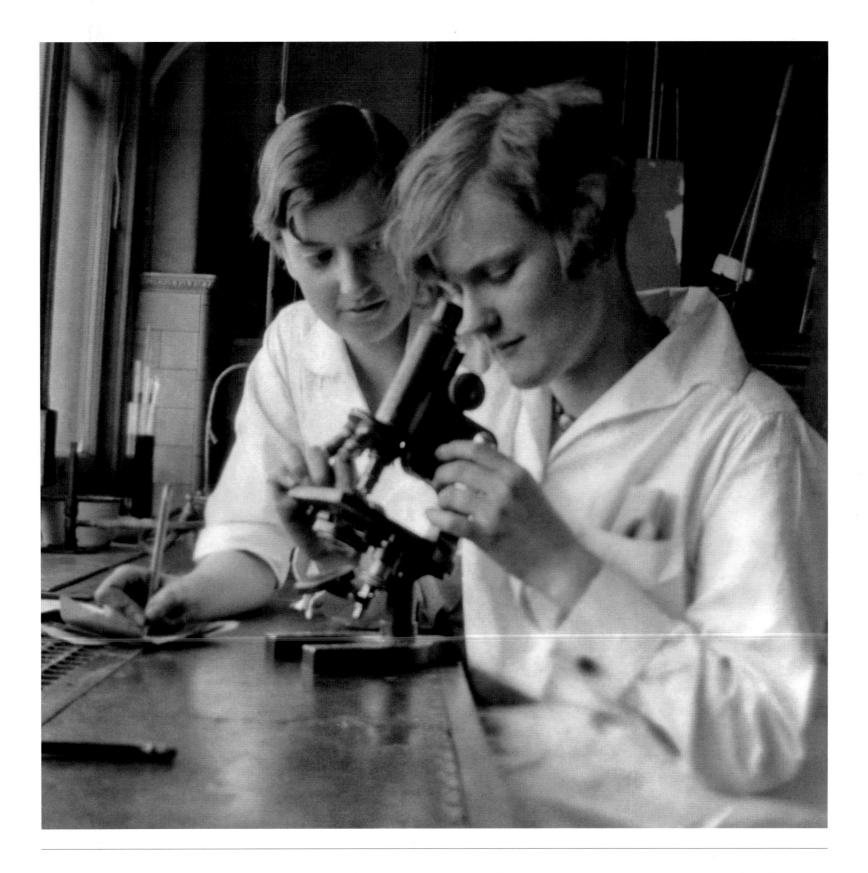

The great contribution we can make is to prepare the oncoming generations to think that they can, and will, think for themselves.

—DR. CHARLIE MAYO

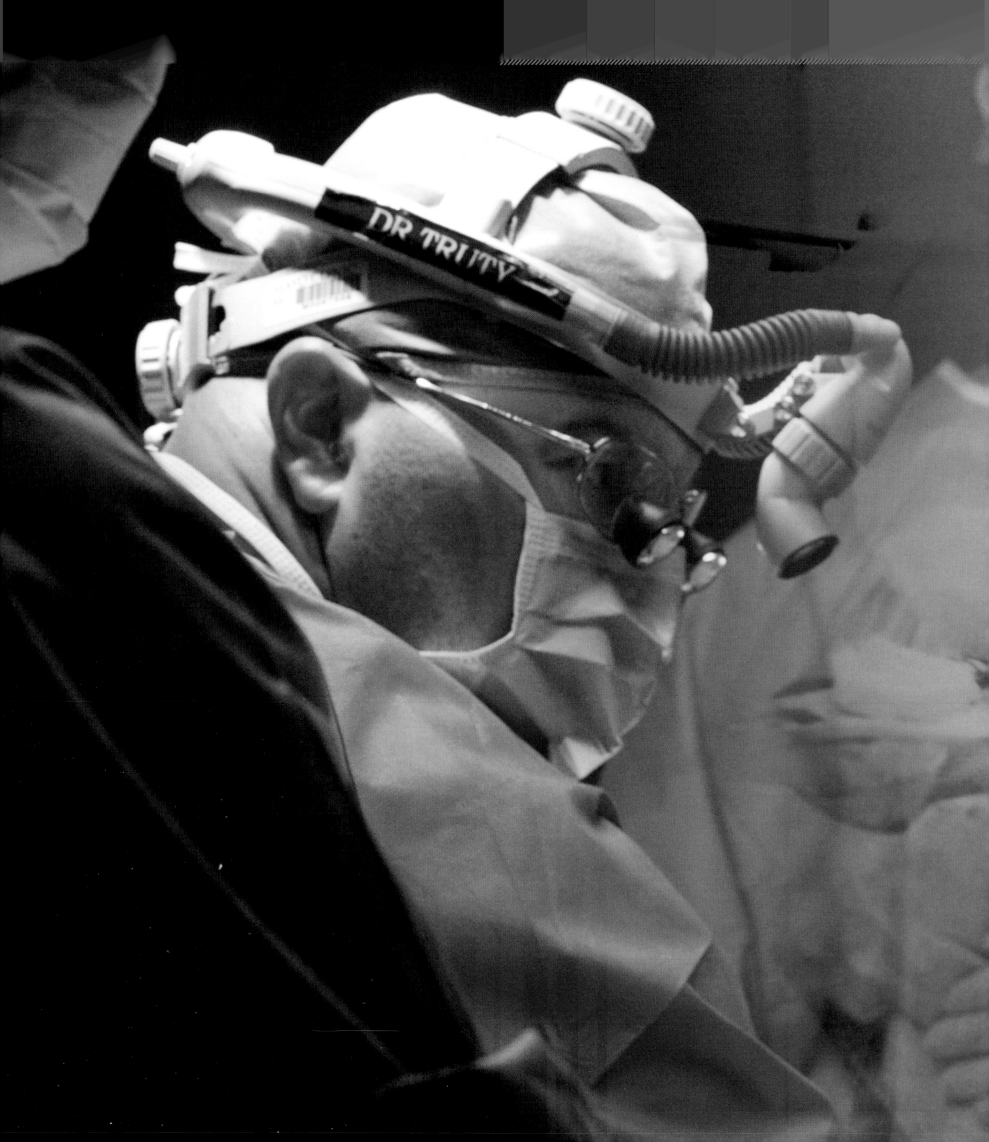

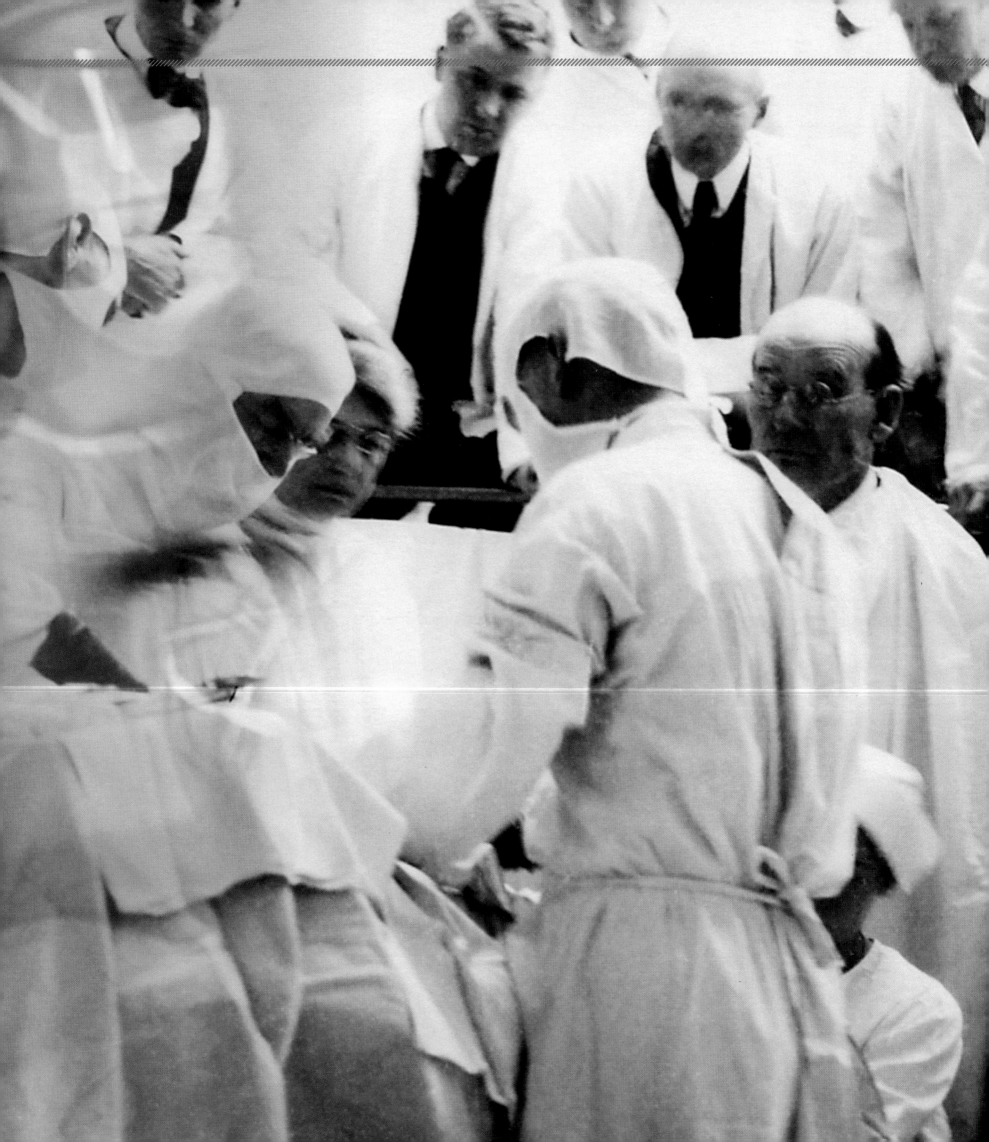

DIAGNOSIS: *PANCREATIC CANCER*

KARL SCHENK (Mission Hill, SD): When you've been given the diagnosis of pancreatic cancer, you know in the back of your mind it's a death sentence. It's like being hit by a freight train and all your senses are gone. You can't hear anything over the noise of the train; you can't feel anything. You only know you're 49 years old and you have four kids at home. And then you start looking for answers. There's a lot of pessimism in the medical community regarding pancreatic cancer. It was pretty clear I needed to get my affairs in order. You have two options: do nothing and die or take a chance on living. The choice is easy. You just need a physician, a surgeon, that's willing to have that same mind-set.

MARK TRUTY, M.D. (Mayo Clinic surgical oncologist): Mr. Schenk came to me with a very advanced pancreas cancer. His tumor was essentially involving all the critical major blood vessels in his abdomen. By any standard definition he would never be a surgical candidate.

KS: The normal protocol for pancreatic cancer is to do the surgery first, and then treat with chemotherapy. The protocols here at Mayo are reversed, and they're having much better results.

MT: I do tend to take the patients that are denied care elsewhere because they are deemed "nonsurgical." We're delivering specific therapies that are currently available in the right dose. Knowing when to stop, when to move on to the next therapy. In the end, he ended up with an operation that's never been done before—with an outstanding result. It was met with a lot of skepticism. That's the one thing that's always surprised me—in medicine and even cancer in general: When you want to introduce a new viewpoint, there's a lot of pushback from people who have been doing it a certain way for many decades.

KS: Currently I am in remission. They can find no cancer in my body at this time. I think Dr. Truty got it, and I've got another twenty-five, thirty years in front of me for sure. Here at Mayo you are a person. When no one else believed, when no one else was giving me options, Mark wouldn't give up. If nothing else, even if your time is limited, you can walk away from Mayo with hope.

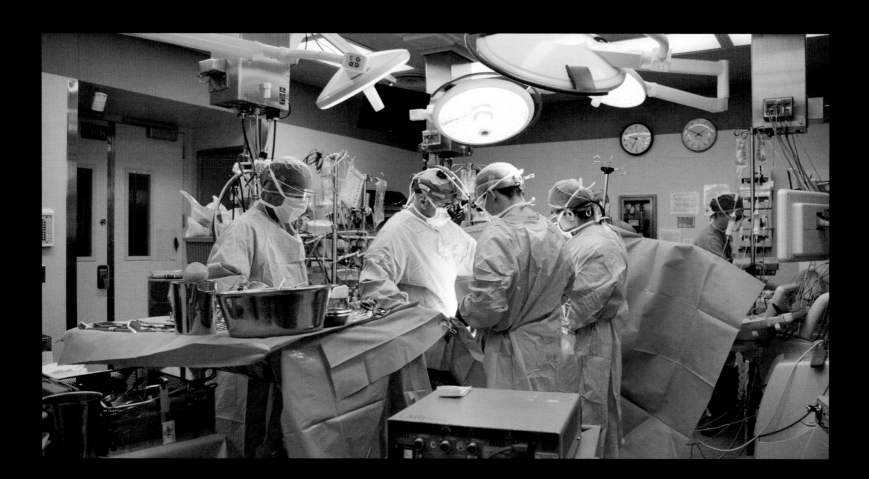

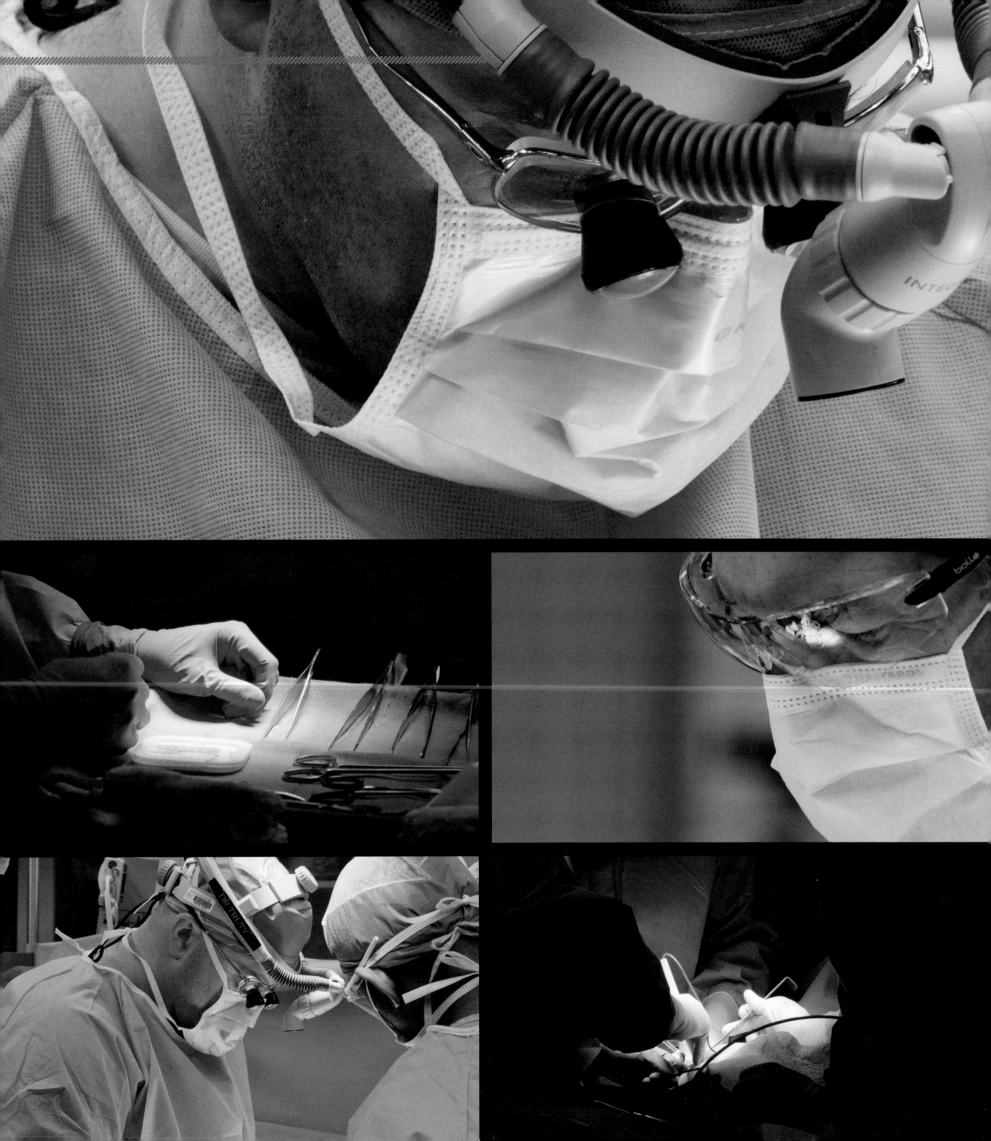

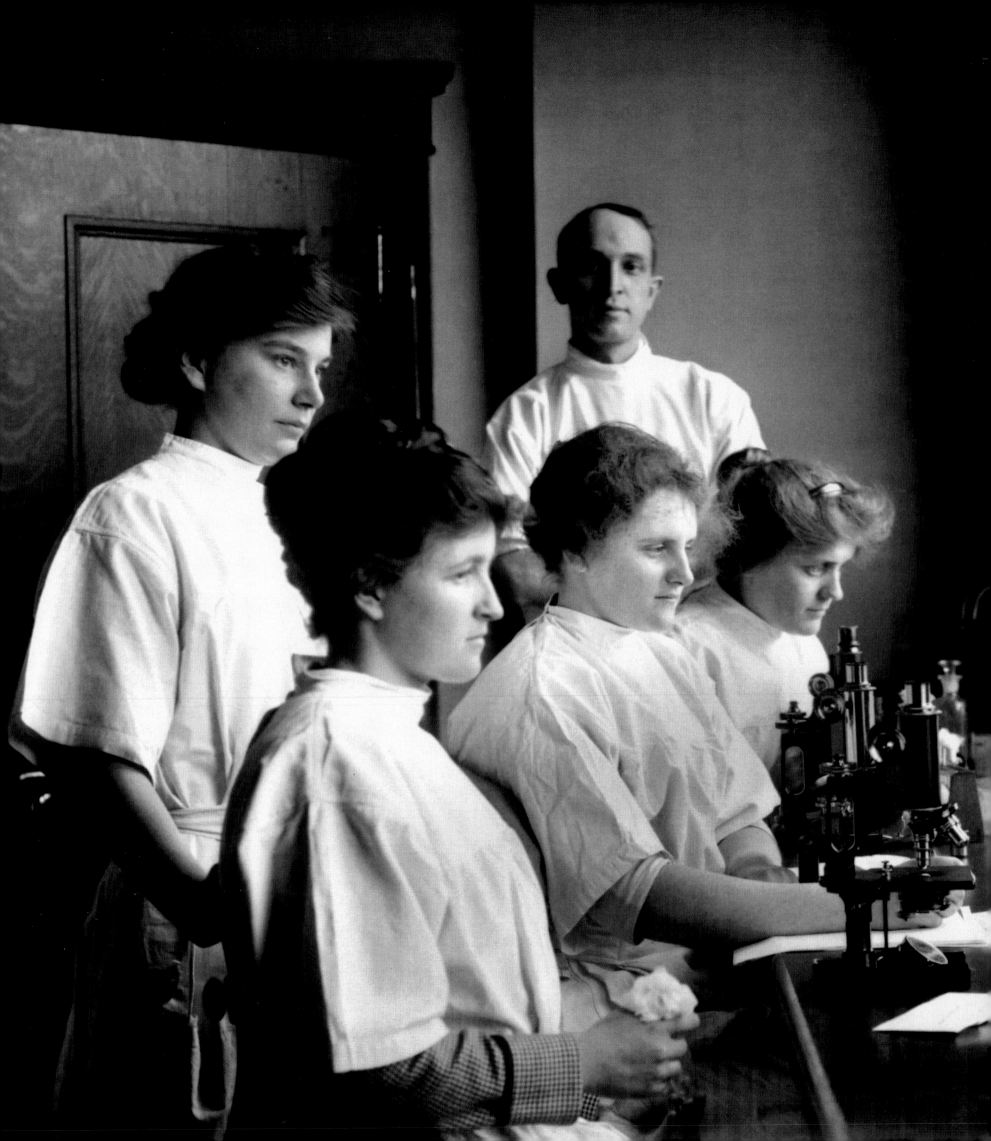

MEDICAL DEMOCRACY

My brother and I had paid for our homes. Our clinic was on its feet. Patients kept coming. Our theories seemed to be working out. Money began to pile up. To us it seemed to be more money than any two men had any right to have. That money seemed, somehow, like holy money to us....[It] had to go back into the service of the humanity that had paid it to us.

—DR. WILL MAYO

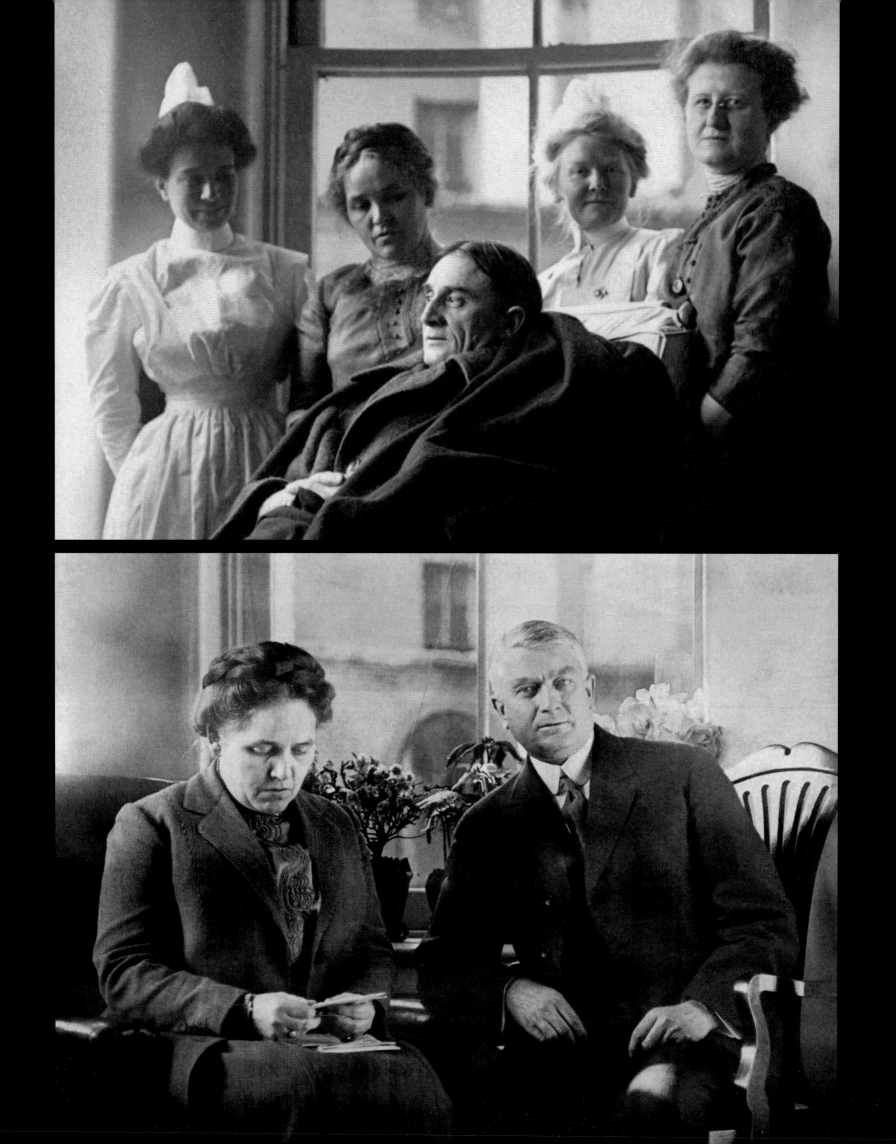

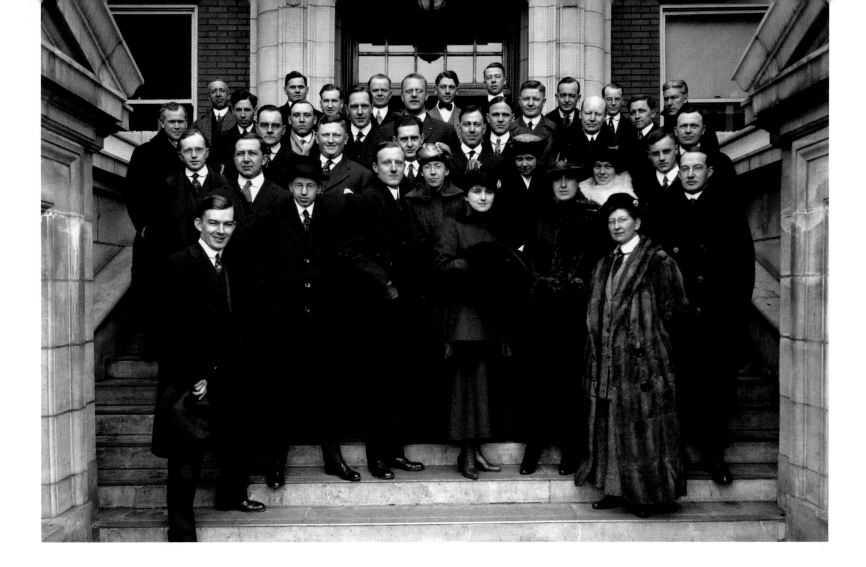

After the United States entered the Great War in 1917, a Mayo Unit was set up in France near the Belgian border, where they cared for more than 7,000 soldiers. Those left behind in Rochester struggled under the increased workload. Things got worse when the Spanish influenza broke out in the fall of 1918. It ultimately killed millions more than the World War.

Dr. Charlie developed a serious case of pneumonia and Dr. Will had jaundice so severe that he suspected it was liver cancer. Both survived, but the experiences made them even more aware of the need to prepare for a time when they could no longer lead the Clinic.

On October 8, 1919, having set aside enough to support their families, Dr. Will, Dr. Charlie, and their wives transferred a significant portion of their personal savings, along with all Mayo Clinic assets and future earnings, to a trust called the Mayo Properties Association. They further stipulated that from then on, all proceeds beyond operating expenses would go to education, research, and patient care.

The Clinic would be run by a Board of Governors, composed almost entirely of Mayo doctors.

"We have in this way," Dr. Will said, "established a medical democracy."

The Mayos also insisted that they, their partners, and all future Mayo physicians would be on salary and would not profit personally from the proceeds of the practice.

> They wanted to make sure that they turned over all the assets to the greater good. If it remained privately owned, money would become part of the dynamics, and take away from the mission. The family had to let go of the authority it had over the practice. That meant all generations would also forfeit that, and if they would have a place in the institution, it would be earned.
>
> —LILLI MAYO WEIVODA, GREAT-GRANDDAUGHTER OF DR. CHARLIE MAYO, ROCHESTER, MN

Opposite, top to bottom: Dr. Charlie; Dr. Will and Hattie Mayo

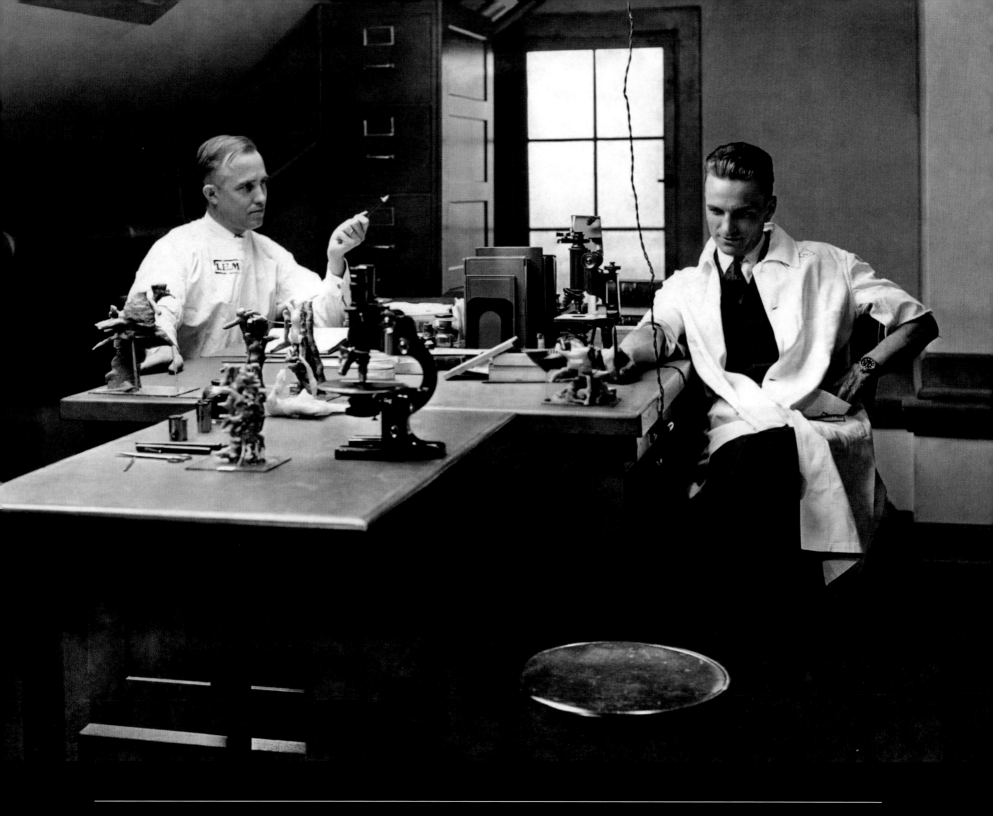

Will and Charlie's idea about putting the faculty members on salaries was brilliant in many ways. In private practice, it's a fee-for-service situation, so if you see more patients, you make more money. That leads some physicians to see more patients in a day, and that leads to them being able to spend less time with the patient. The Mayo physicians were going to get paid the same regardless of whether they ordered the test or referred the patients for surgery.

—CHRISTOPHER BOES, M.D., MAYO CLINIC NEUROLOGIST

We choose to be here because we value this teamwork and this environment over our own compensation. This place tends to select people who want to have that type of teamwork.

**—DEBORAH RHODES, M.D.,
MAYO CLINIC INTERNIST**

There will never be a decision made about patient care that benefits the physician. It's always about the patient. And that helps us keep pure, our decisions going forward, that the collective whole is better than the sum from any individual. At Mayo Clinic you are never alone in your efforts to find an answer to that patient's problem.

**—JOHN NOSEWORTHY, M.D.,
PRESIDENT AND CEO, MAYO CLINIC**

Mayo Clinic is an engineering wonder. If you go to Mayo, you all of a sudden find this highly integrated and engineered system, like a well-oiled machine, and it comes from Plummer's vision and the Mayos' vision; it comes from the idea that all these pieces that were spread out are part of the same clockwork.

—SIDDHARTHA MUKHERJEE, M.D., PH.D., ONCOLOGIST, AUTHOR, COLUMBIA UNIVERSITY

By 1920, only a quarter of the medical staff at Mayo Clinic were surgeons. The rest were physicians and scientists who not only examined and diagnosed patients, but also researched the underlying causes of disease in order to improve surgical outcomes and develop nonsurgical treatments. It was the rapidly growing field of internal medicine—and Mayo Clinic was at the forefront:

- Henry Plummer and Walter Boothby's discovery in 1923 of how to treat enlarged thyroid glands with iodine before surgery greatly reduced mortality rates.

- Dr. Albert Broders made a major contribution to cancer diagnosis by developing a technique for grading tumors—based on how likely the mutated cells were to spread.

- In 1922, Dr. Russell Wilder and four colleagues conducted one of the earliest clinical trials of insulin. Within a year, more than 20,000 diabetic patients in the United States were being treated successfully.

When the patients really started an influx to the community, they saw that there was a need for additional hotels and restaurants, and the community really embraced Mayo Clinic.

—RENEE ZIEMER, MAYO CLINIC HISTORIAN

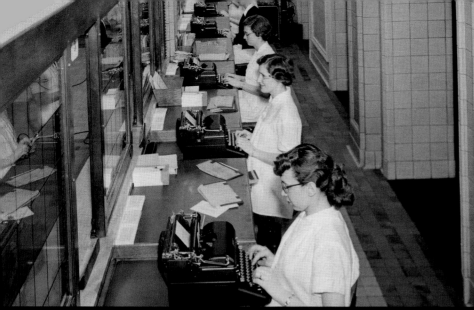

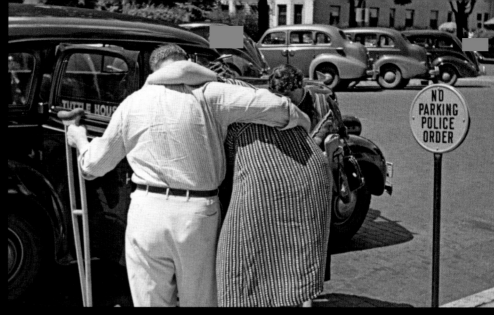

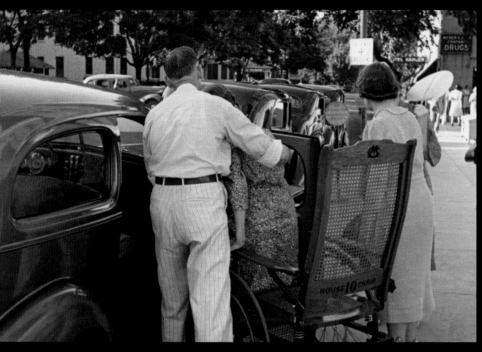

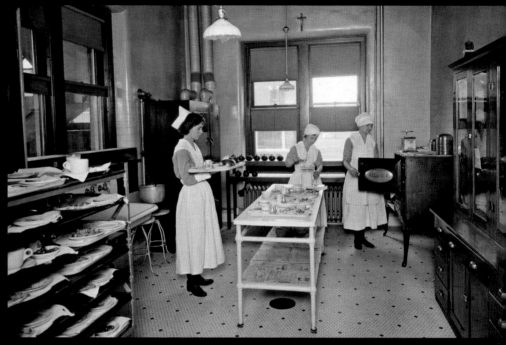

It's the person who opens the door, it's the person who meets them in the hallways, it's the person who says, "You look lost; can I help you find your way?" It's the desk attendant, it's the secretary, it's the custodian, it's pervasive.

—JOHN NOSEWORTHY, M.D., PRESIDENT AND CEO, MAYO CLINIC

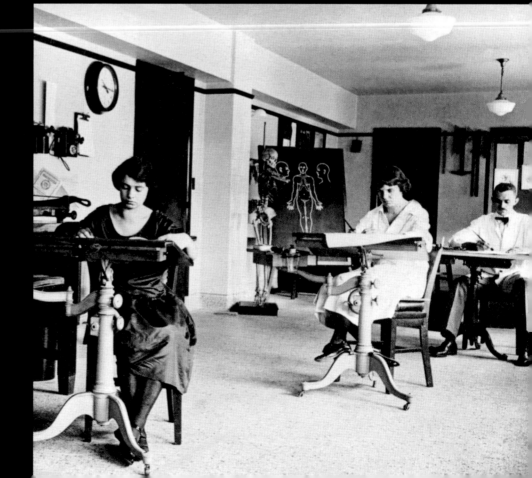

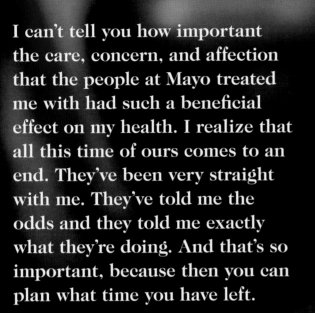

I can't tell you how important the care, concern, and affection that the people at Mayo treated me with had such a beneficial effect on my health. I realize that all this time of ours comes to an end. They've been very straight with me. They've told me the odds and they told me exactly what they're doing. And that's so important, because then you can plan what time you have left.

—JOHN MCCAIN, PATIENT, PHOENIX, AZ

By the mid-1920s, more than 60,000 patients were arriving at Mayo Clinic every year. In response, Saint Marys built an impressive new surgical pavilion. At the same time, local businessman John Kahler constructed several innovative hotel-hospitals that could accommodate the massive influx of patients and their families. Eventually, Kahler's health-care facilities would evolve into a new nonprofit hospital called Rochester Methodist.

Mayo Clinic was overwhelmed, too. Henry Plummer agreed to oversee yet another expansion project. Completed in 1928, the $3 million, seventeen-story Plummer Building was the tallest in the state. Constructed of limestone and brick, it featured marble from France, Germany, and Italy; hand-carved ornamental designs; two solid bronze doors; and an 18-ton, 23-bell carillon.

Plummer devised an ingenious series of lifts to automatically deliver medical records to designated floors before patients arrived for their appointments. He also developed an array of signal lights outside the exam rooms so nurses could track the status of every appointment. There was even a system of pneumatic tubes to send medical records and specimens between Mayo Clinic and Saint Marys Hospital—a mile away.

The Mayos insisted on a degree of distinction in Mayo Clinic buildings. For many patients, this will be their encounter with beautiful architecture and design and art. It's so important to put them in a frame of mind of healing. So fast-forward to Cesar Pelli, the designer of the Gonda Building: He said healing begins when you walk in the door, before you ever see your doctor, you have this sense of, *I've come to a good place*. All of this is part of the healing mission of Mayo.

—MATTHEW DACY, MAYO CLINIC HISTORIAN

It's a challenging point in our history that we have to acknowledge. That was the decision that was made because that was the culture of our time. The decisions that we make are ultimately about the patient, but if you are not serving the staff the same way, then you ultimately don't serve those patients. We just have to learn from things that we've done in the past, and get to a new point for our future.

—JOHN WALD, M.D., MAYO CLINIC
NEURORADIOLOGIST

But for all its innovation and success, Mayo Clinic is not a perfect place. Access is problematic. Diseases are relentless, their cures elusive. Mistakes are made. Patients are misdiagnosed. Treatments fail. People die.

Occasionally, Mayo's emphasis on putting the patient first has led to decisions in direct conflict with its original values. Although Mayo Clinic welcomed patients of all races and regularly invited minority doctors as distinguished guests, they—as at most hospitals across the country—were not allowed to treat white patients, who might not be comfortable with a black doctor.

There wouldn't be an African-American physician on staff until 1979.

Every physician has a personal private cemetery at the back of their minds. It's a graveyard of all the previous patients they failed, and it's a place that we all go to reflect upon our shortcomings and try to decide, How do we improve upon this?

—MARK TRUTY, M.D.,
MAYO CLINIC SURGICAL
ONCOLOGIST

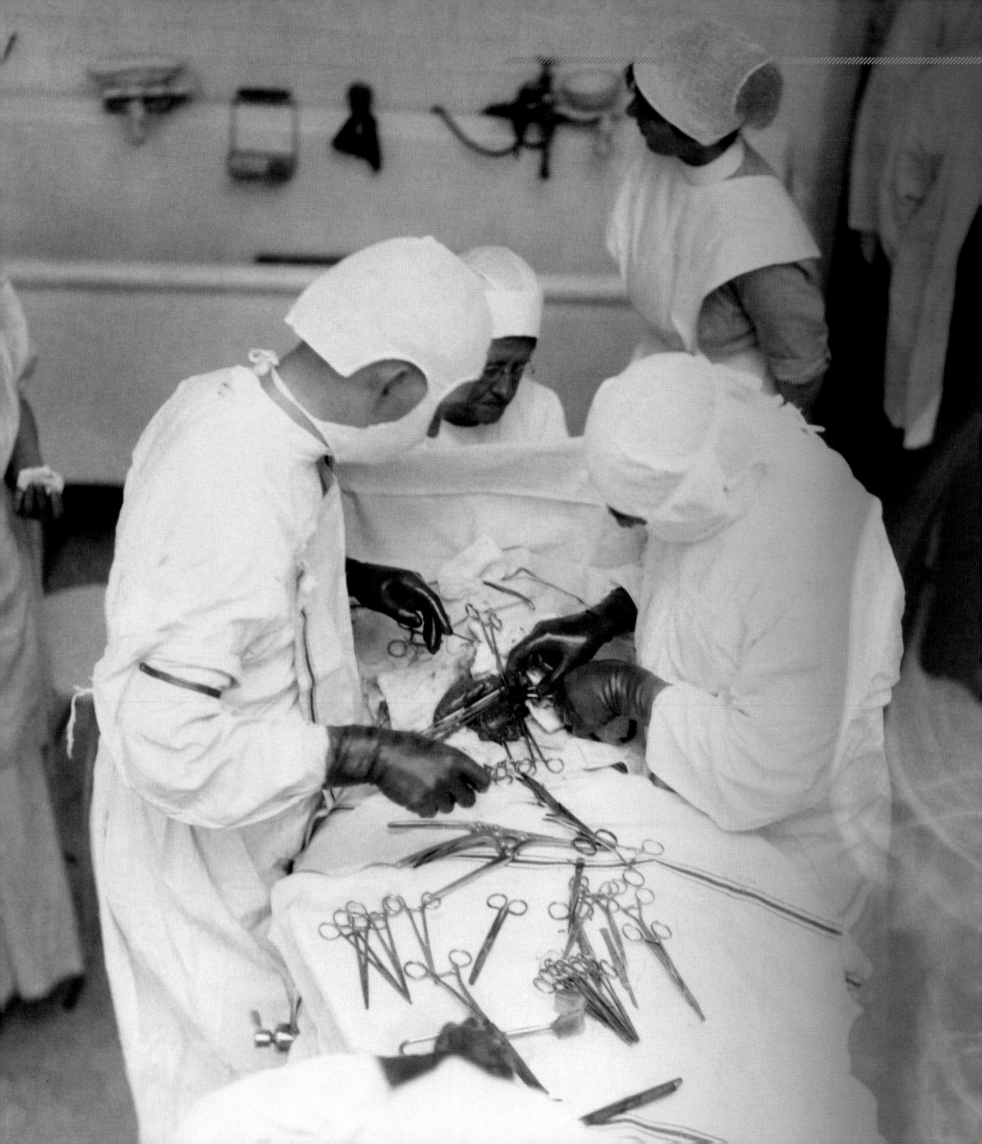

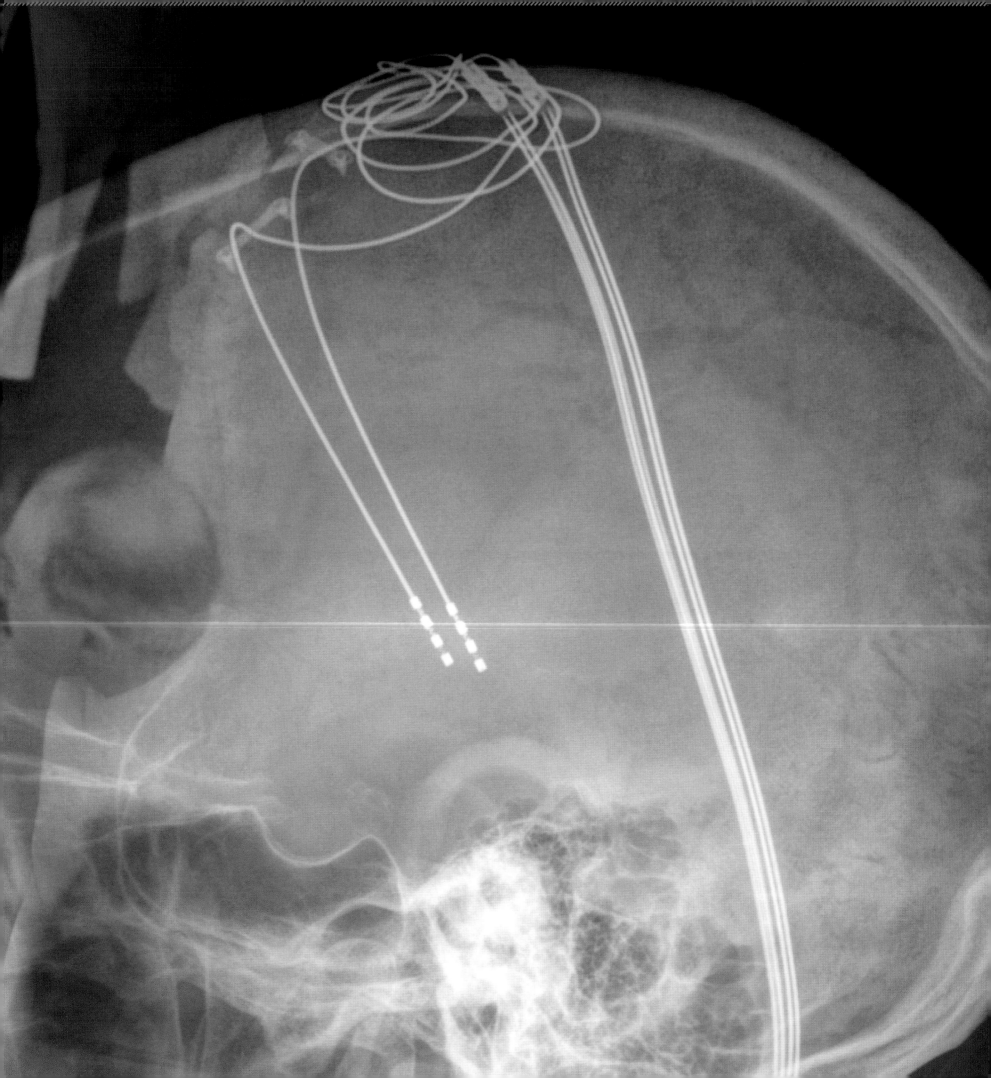

COLLABORATION

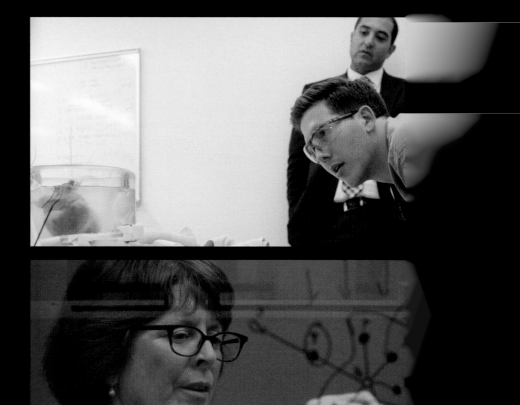

RAFAEL SIERRA, M.D. (Mayo Clinic orthopedic surgeon): In many institutions there are researchers, and there are clinicians, and they can both be excellent, but there are very few places where they both come together.

ATTA BEHFAR, M.D., Ph.D. (Mayo Clinic cardiologist): To be both a physician and scientist, if we can identify disease at its purest form, we'll be able to, in a very minimally invasive way, dramatically change the life course of an individual.

RS: Atta has been doing some innovative work in cardiac regeneration in regards to heart failure. And that is what we've also used as our bridge to work in my field, which is in orthopedics. We take cells from an individual and also try to regenerate bone.

JUDY BOUGHEY, M.D. (Mayo Clinic breast surgical oncologist): I've enjoyed some research on evaluating the role of surgery, in particular surgery of the lymph nodes, in terms of patients with breast cancer.

HEIDI NELSON, M.D. (Mayo Clinic general surgeon): I think Mayo Clinic has been dedicated to research since the founders themselves were. The Mayo brothers wrote about the possible role of germs in cancer. And that's come to be true.

AB: Will and Charlie, setting up the concept of investigation as part of your practice, created a culture at Mayo, right from its origins. If we have a careful consideration of the patients' welfare in mind, and if we show scientifically the evidence for our discovery, then it's an irrefutable finding. That's when true innovation occurs in medicine.

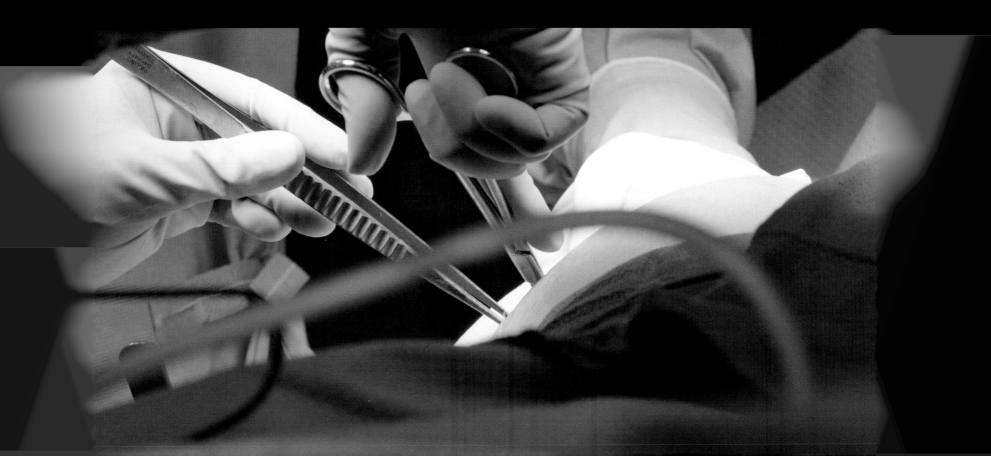

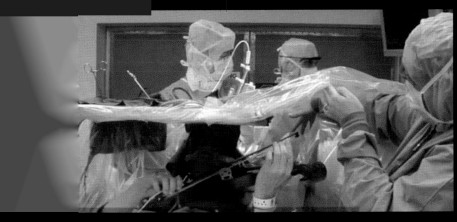

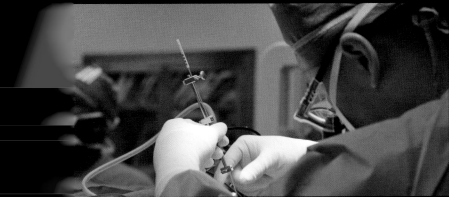

TREATMENT: DEEP BRAIN STIMULATION

ROGER FRISCH (Minneapolis, MN): The first time I noticed something was not quite right, the rehearsal started, and I started drawing a very slow bow and, for the first time ever, I noticed a little tiny shake in my bow arm—the arm that needs to have absolute perfect control. As a musician, that's when you start panicking. I must have gone to about fifteen different doctors, and no one could really come up with an answer. I considered the possibility this was the end of my career.

KENDALL LEE, M.D., Ph.D. (Mayo Clinic neurosurgeon): He started to play his violin, and it was clear that he couldn't play. And he said, "Can you help me with this?"

RF: Dr. Lee said, "I've been working on a technique that involves drilling a hole in your head." I had one reaction: No one is ever drilling a hole in my head. But after three months of the tremor getting worse and worse, someone drilling a hole in my head maybe wasn't such a bad idea.

KL: Deep brain stimulation is a technique where we can target anywhere in the brain with an electrode, and stimulate that area of the brain. What we find, amazingly, is that in our patients with tremor, we can actually make those symptoms go away.

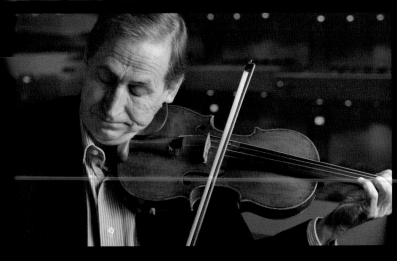

RF: I was fully awake because they needed me to play violin during the surgery. Dr. Lee inserted the first lead and I started to play and the tremor was much better, but it wasn't good enough to play professionally. They inserted the second lead, and I drew a bow and it was perfectly steady. They give me this little control switch which I always think is like a garage door opener, but I can actually turn myself on and off. It says I'm off now, and if you wait about five seconds, then it really does kick in almost right away. As hard as I try, that's as smooth as I get, and you can see the bow just shaking just me holding it. So now I'm back on again. And wait about five seconds...

KL: We often say in the lab, *Patients are waiting.* And so we have to discover the new cures. Today. We're on a mission to help the patient in a timely fashion. This is not a theoretical academic exercise. We want the cure because we see the patient suffering today.

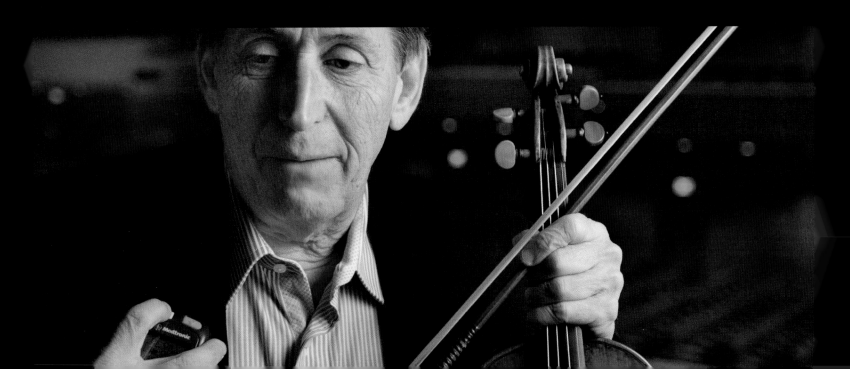

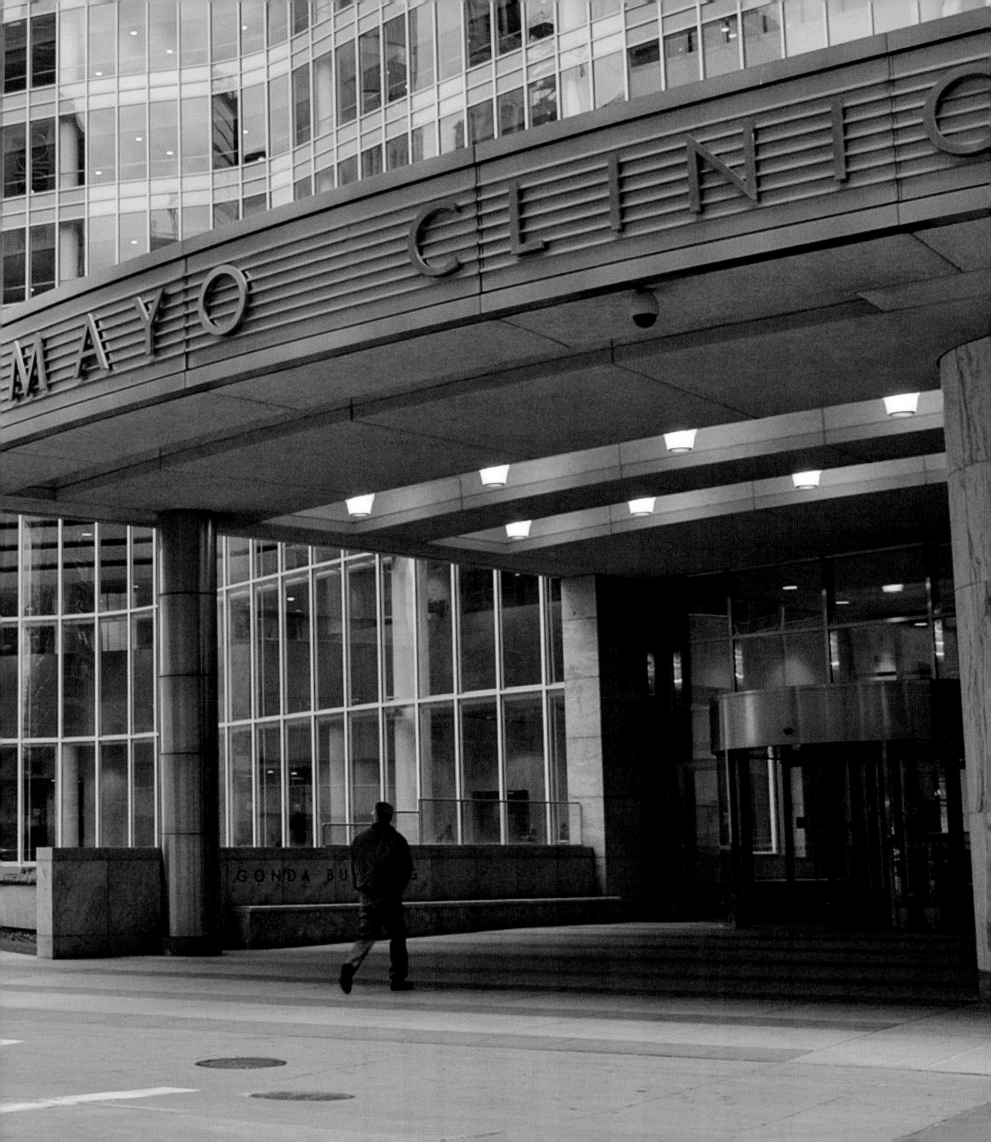

CHAPTER SEVEN

AN ENDURING LEGACY

Medicine is both an art and a science, and both make appeal to the true physician.

—DR. CHARLIE MAYO

> I think the Mayos thought about the future all the time. I don't think they ever looked back over their shoulders. I think it was always, "I'll deal with what I've got in front of me, but how do I face the next thing, and what is the next thing?"
>
> **—LILLI MAYO WEIVODA, GREAT-GRANDDAUGHTER OF DR. CHARLIE MAYO, ROCHESTER, MN**

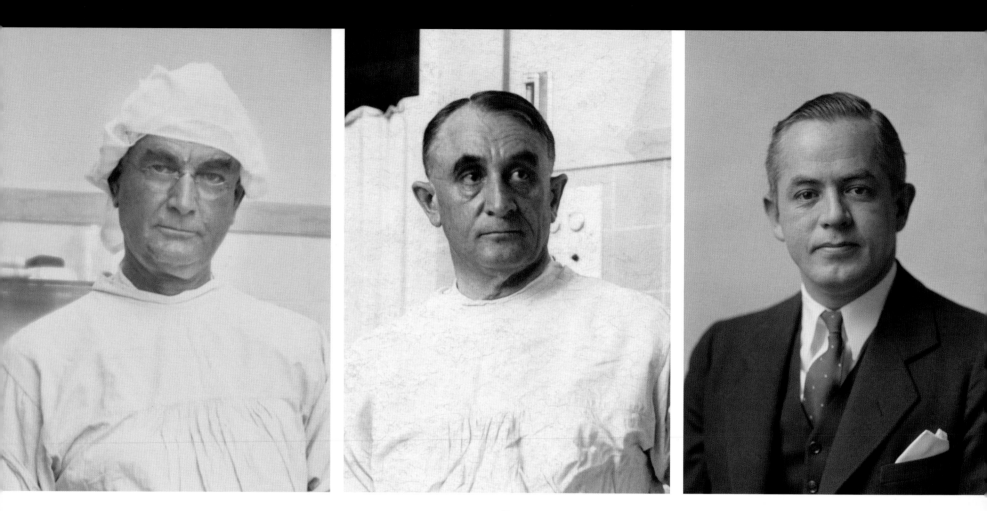

One day in 1928, Dr. Will arrived at his office and told his secretary that he had just performed his last operation. He had developed a slight tremor in his hands. When she protested, he explained, "I want to stop while I'm still good."

Meanwhile, Dr. Charlie's son, known as Dr. Chuck, had received his medical degree and was looking forward to working with his father, just as young Charlie and Will had worked side by side with their father.

On Dr. Chuck's very first day as surgical assistant, his father suffered a dizzy spell. It turned out to be the first of a series of minor strokes. Dr. Charlie's surgical days were over, too.

I had been dreaming for years... of being his first assistant, amazing and impressing him with my skill. I thought, I suppose, that it would draw us together. But fate gave me only that one morning to prove myself.

—CHARLES W. MAYO, M.D.

Left to right: Dr. Will, Dr. Charlie, Dr. Chuck
Opposite, second from top: Dr. Will, Dr. Charlie, and FDR
Opposite, bottom: Sister Joseph Dempsey and FDR

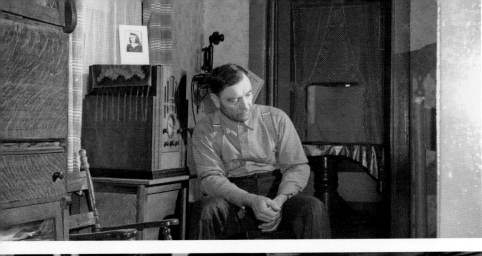

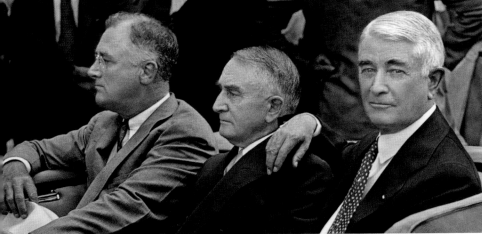

The Great Depression tested Mayo Clinic like no other event. Doctors and staff accepted pay cuts to minimize layoffs. The Clinic printed "Mayo money" in case employees needed help paying for rent and food. No one was turned away because of their inability to pay, but the number of patients seeking treatment fell dramatically.

At Saint Marys, the situation was even more precarious. But having made vows of poverty, the Sisters knew how to adapt. They raised turkeys and chickens, harvested acres of fruits and vegetables, and pasteurized almost a quarter of a million gallons of milk a year—which they not only used to feed their patients, but also shared with the many needy people who arrived at their door begging for food.

The reduced patient loads during the Depression did give doctors time to do experiments they had been putting off. Edward Kendall and Philip Hench began work that would lead to the discovery of cortisone, for which they would be awarded a Nobel Prize. Dr. Hugh Butt discovered that vitamin K could save the lives of patients with jaundice. And Dr. John Lundy established one of the nation's first blood banks.

On Wednesday, August 8, 1934, with temperatures in the nineties, 75,000 people—three times the city's population—gathered along Broadway to see President Franklin D. Roosevelt ride with Dr. Will and Dr. Charlie from the train station through town.

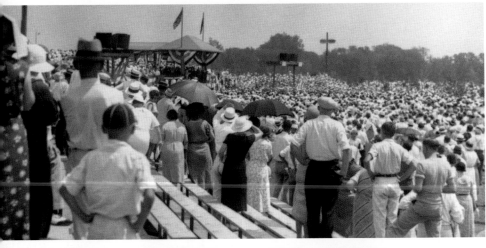

FDR had come to present the Mayos with an award from the American Legion in honor of their service to the country, which included providing free care to World War I veterans. During his visit, Roosevelt laid a wreath at the grave of W.W. Mayo, and stopped at Saint Marys, where Sister Joseph Dempsey came alongside his car and clasped the President's hands.

The town had been preparing for weeks. A portable stage with a hidden ramp had been built so the President could reach the platform without the crowd seeing the metal braces on his legs, which were crippled by polio. His ten-minute tribute to the Mayo brothers was broadcast on radio throughout the country.

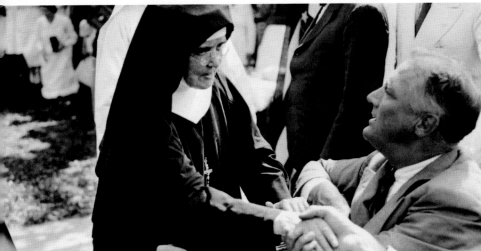

I hope that the people of Minnesota and of Rochester will not feel limited in their pride of possession when the nation which I have the honor to represent claims the right to call Dr. Will and Dr. Charlie by the good word of "neighbor."

—FRANKLIN DELANO ROOSEVELT, PRESIDENT, UNITED STATES

CLAIRE W RICHARDS

1990 – 2014

Dear Dr. Markovic, I think it's clear that I'm reaching the end of my road. Our gratitude to you and the Mayo Clinic is beyond words....You always have believed in me and my future, despite the unbearable odds that have been against us....You gave me the gift of time, of months of life that I otherwise wouldn't have had....Countless times you gave my family and I hope when we had none....You are an inspiration and a godsend to your patients.

CLAIRE RICHARDS, PATIENT, MINNEAPOLIS, MN

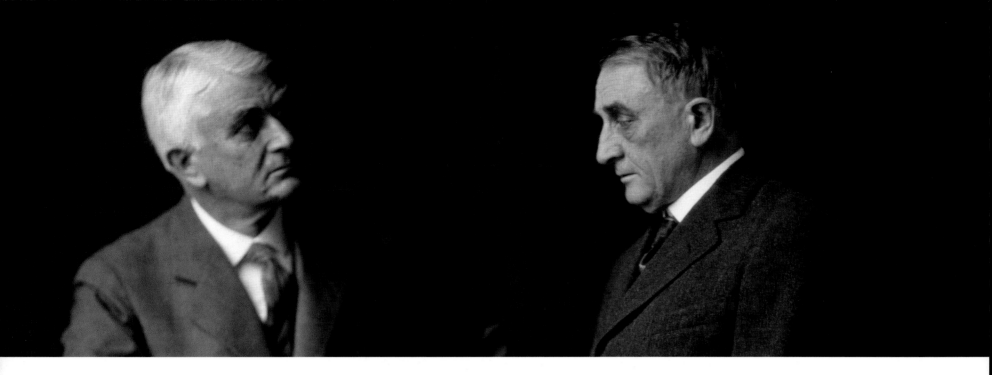

Will and Charlie Mayo spent much of the winter in side-by-side adobe houses they had built in Tucson, Arizona. At 8 every morning, they would meet at Charlie's house to review news from the Clinic. "Well, well," Charlie once said, "this is quite a comedown for us, Will. They're doing better now that we're away."

In 1938, Mayo Clinic officially treated its one-millionth patient. But there would be little else to celebrate. Sister Joseph, the resourceful 82-year-old leader of Saint Marys Hospital for four decades, had retired. She could still be found visiting patients at Saint Marys—particularly children, the poor, and alcoholics. But early the next spring she came down with pneumonia and died on March 29, 1939, surrounded by her Franciscan Sisters.

In April, Dr. Will began having stomach pains. An X-ray showed it was cancer. The man who had operated on so many abdominal tumors now had a tumor of his own removed by a Mayo surgical team. Will seemed to be recovering, but then Charlie came down with a serious case of pneumonia.

Granddaddy was sitting straight up in a high-back rose-colored chair. …His glasses had slipped low on his nose, and his mouth allowed soft air to escape. Granny was leaning over him…. "Isn't he beautiful?" she said. "Isn't he the most handsome man?" I asked her what she was doing. She said she was memorizing his face "in case he leaves me first—I want to remember what he looks like."

—CHARLES H. MAYO, II, M.D., GRANDSON OF DR. CHARLIE MAYO

Dr. Charlie died on May 26, 1939.

Not long after Father died, Uncle Will noted with professional interest that he was becoming jaundiced. He diagnosed it at once as metastasis in his liver. He went about his death in the same practical, crisp manner, with no self-pity. He summoned the family: "I've had a good life, and this is all right. I'm not going to have any further medication except some morphine for the pain. I'll say goodbye to you now."

—CHARLES W. MAYO, M.D., SON OF DR. CHARLIE MAYO

On July 28, Dr. Will died.

It must have been a tremendously solemn time at Mayo Clinic. To lose those three. Those three leaders. An awful lot of people believed that when the Mayo brothers died, the Clinic would go into decline. And it didn't. Others believed that as change occurred in society, the need for the Mayo Clinic and its success would go into decline, and none of that happened. The Clinic has grown and has flourished long after the Mayo brothers left this earth.

—JOHN NOSEWORTHY, M.D., PRESIDENT AND CEO, MAYO CLINIC

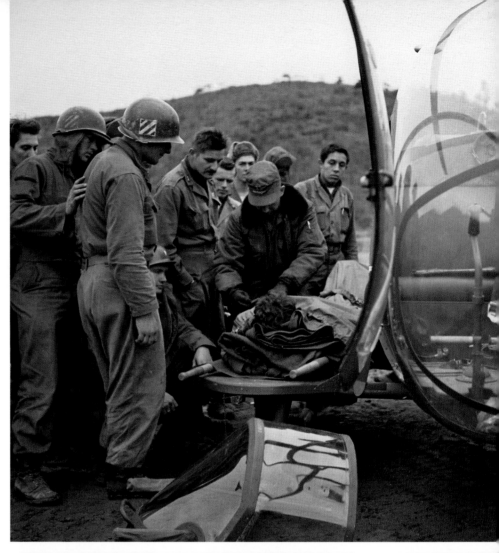

Mayo Clinic sponsored several medical teams during the Second World War, including one in the Philippines. Led by Charlie's son Dr. Chuck, it built hospitals in the jungle where they treated both Allied and Japanese soldiers.

In the new Medical Sciences Building, a top-secret Aeromedical Unit developed an inflatable G-suit that protected Allied pilots from blacking out on steep dives. The Aeromedical Unit had cost the Mayo Clinic $2 million. Mayo Clinic charged the United States government one dollar.

In the years ahead, Mayo doctors and nurses would help assemble MASH units for the Korean War, devise plans to deal with potential mass casualties during the Cold War, and, after 9/11, developed a rapid test to diagnose anthrax.

Mayo doctors also used the first CT scanner in the country, pioneered the use of computers in operating rooms, performed the first series of successful surgeries using a heart–lung bypass machine, and developed one of the first combined liver–heart transplant programs. Mayo Clinic has also helped the medical community accelerate the pace of stem cell, gene-based, and other individualized therapies.

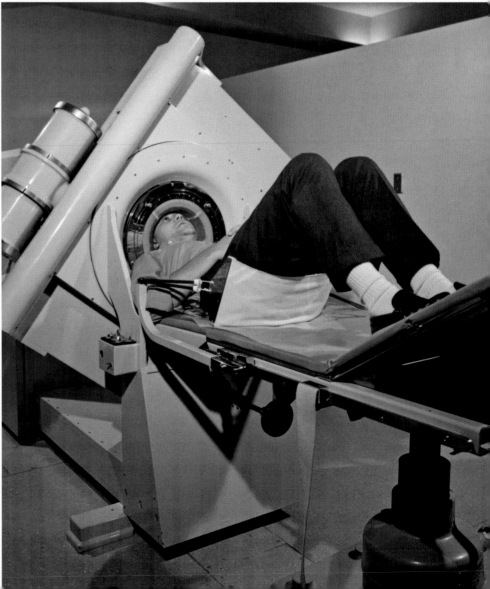

> The greatest asset of a nation is the health of its people. The medical profession can be the greatest factor for good in America. Our failures as a profession are the failures of individualism, the result of competitive medicine. It must be done by collective effort.
>
> **—DR. WILL MAYO**

The biggest challenge facing Mayo Clinic, and every other hospital and doctor in America, is the issue of cost and administration of health care. For more than fifty years, as the country argued over what it owed its citizens, Mayo Clinic struggled to remain true to the values W.W. had instilled in his sons.

With Medicare and Medicaid, everybody was supposed to have good health insurance. Well, that didn't actually work out as planned. There were supposed to be health maintenance organizations. That didn't work well. There was supposed to be regional health planning. And that didn't work. Most recently we've had this consumer-oriented movement—competition will bring down costs, we'll make it more efficient. Well, that hasn't worked. One of the messages from Mayo's history is that you can be entrepreneurial and competitive and idealistic and put the patient first all at the same time. And that is the message now that leaders of these organizations all across the country are trying to tackle.

—ROSEMARY A. STEVENS, PH.D., MEDICAL HISTORIAN, WEILL CORNELL MEDICINE

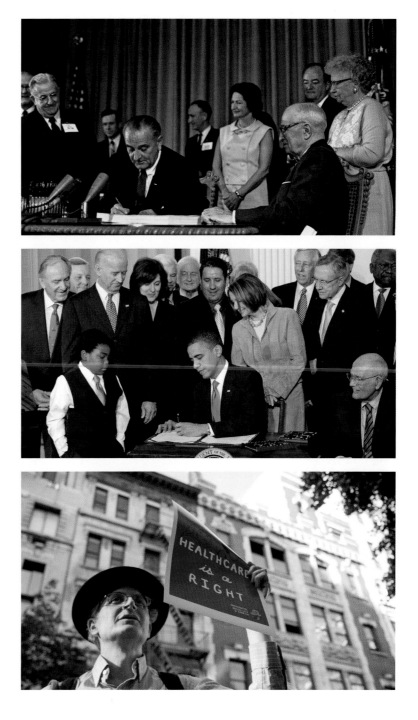

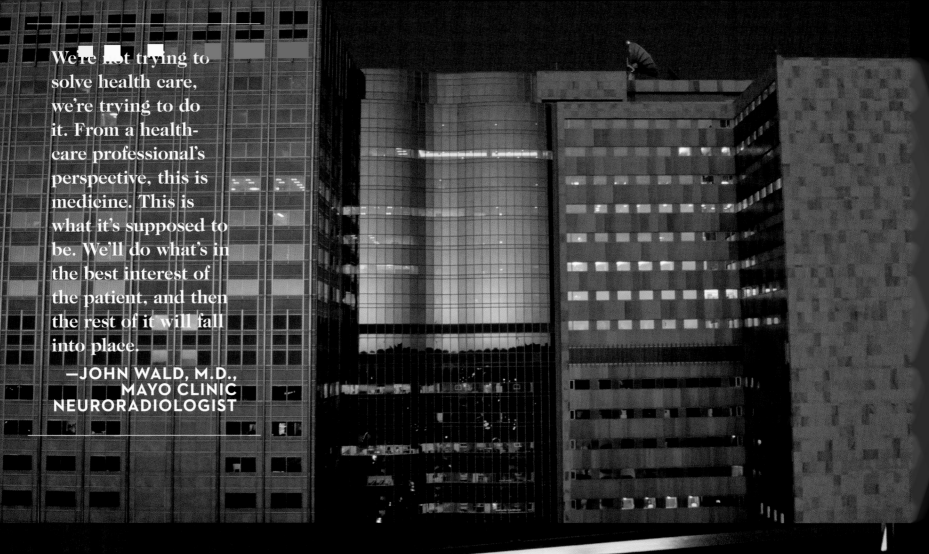

We're not trying to solve health care, we're trying to do it. From a health-care professional's perspective, this is medicine. This is what it's supposed to be. We'll do what's in the best interest of the patient, and then the rest of it will fall into place.

**—JOHN WALD, M.D.,
MAYO CLINIC
NEURORADIOLOGIST**

Mayo Clinic is on a historic pedestal. But it needs to be maintained—not just dusted, like a sculpture on a pedestal, but really maintained—in a way that the physiology of the institution remains active and viable and vital. It's an island of excellent medical care, and that has its problems. How to translate that model into extremely diverse communities has remained a huge challenge.

**—SIDDHARTHA MUKHERJEE, M.D.,
PH.D., ONCOLOGIST, AUTHOR,
COLUMBIA UNIVERSITY**

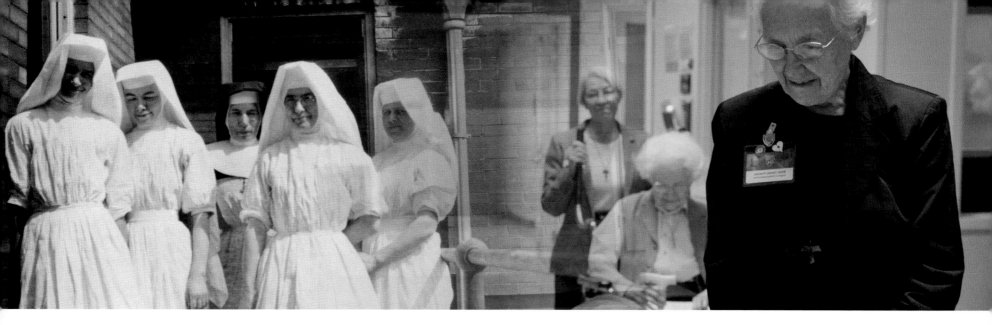

We know who we are with the Sisters, but we don't know who we'd be without them.

—W. EUGENE MAYBERRY, M.D.,
EMERITUS PRESIDENT
AND CEO, MAYO CLINIC

In 1986, Saint Marys Hospital, Mayo Clinic, and Rochester Methodist Hospital merged as an integrated center of medicine with total assets of $1 billion.

Mayo Clinic, which started in a frontier doctor's office in a small Minnesota town, would go on to create medical centers in Jacksonville, Florida, and Scottsdale, Arizona, the regional Mayo Clinic Health System, the Mayo Clinic College of Medicine and Science, and a worldwide network of like-minded hospitals, all dedicated to working together to find new ways to perfect the Mayos' belief that the needs of the patient must always come first.

I look through a half-opened door into the future, full of interest, intriguing beyond my power to describe, but with a full understanding that it is for each generation to solve its own problems and that no man has the wisdom to guide or control the next generation.

—DR. WILL MAYO

... with all the... execution... skilfully fitted, above and... and geared to the roof... foundation... idly-breaking on the... waiting for the lever... to move its sounds and... commence its life and action... with admiration... superiority of the work... man, when... and all... man... So superior man and... works of the... superiority... and beautiful... for the superior... mixture of soil, clay...

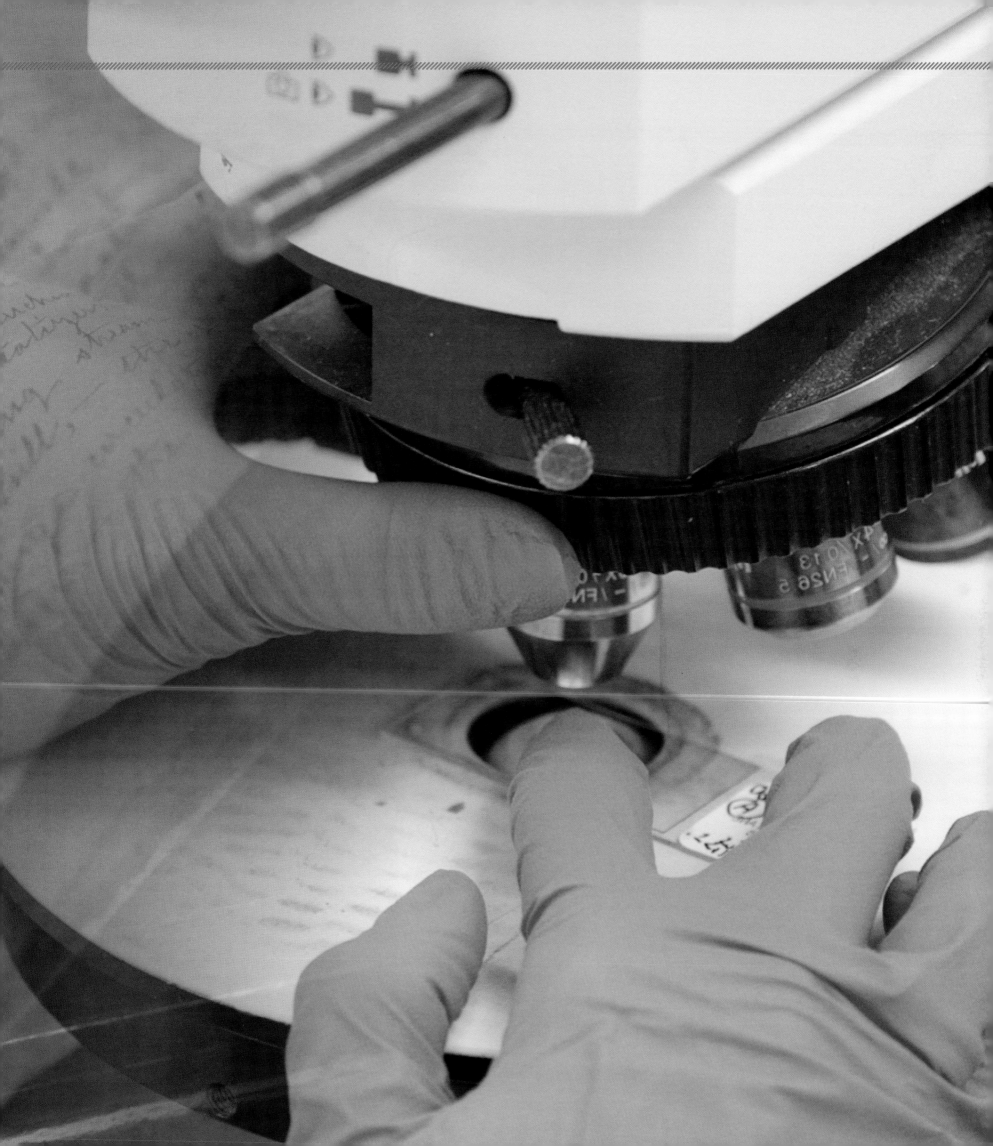

DIAGNOSIS: *LUPUS*

SHANNON LEON (Corn, OK): Over two years, I have seen forty different doctors, and I have been admitted 120 times at my local hospital. And no diagnosis. My liver was failing, and then it went to my kidneys and to my lungs, and then it went to my heart. I have been revived seven times. I always felt like I was passed on from one doctor to another. They did not know what was wrong. They kept me alive, but they never gave me any kind of hope. They said I would not make it past 35.

TIMOTHY NIEWOLD, M.D. (Mayo Clinic rheumatologist): You might see a lung doctor, and then you have to see a kidney doctor somewhere else, but for Shannon, she's thinking it should be one thing that's linking these things together, and I'm not sure anyone's really got that yet. I think most physicians are well meaning and want to try to work within these systems, but it's difficult when everything is so fragmented. This is the health-care system in the United States that we're running into as patients.

SL: Dr. Niewold was the start of my hope. I had many, many tests. The consultation between me and him lasted about two hours. I just told him what was wrong and all my symptoms. He sent me back to the waiting room, and twenty minutes later, exactly twenty minutes, he called me back and gave me a diagnosis. Lupus. Between four and five years and no diagnosis, and twenty minutes with Dr. Niewold. It was like a total miracle.

TN: The pace of medical knowledge isn't going to slow down, and I think it does take more of a distributed mind-set to be able to handle all of that and apply it to patient care.

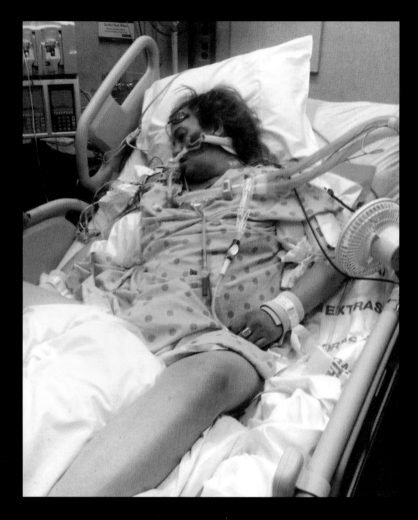

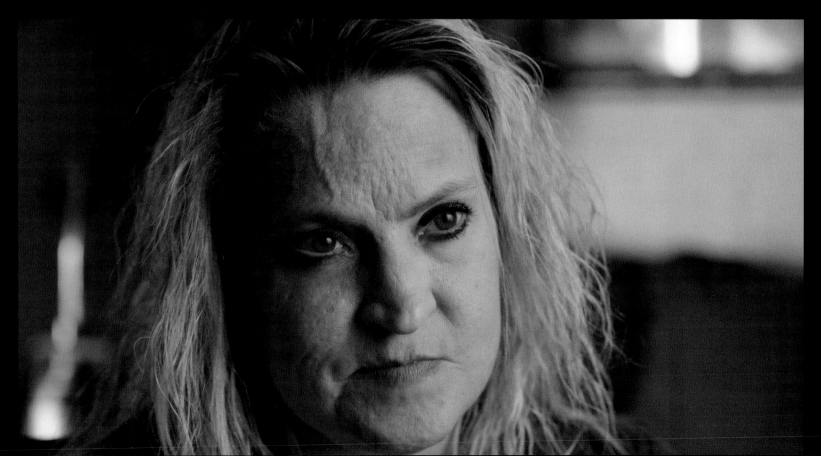

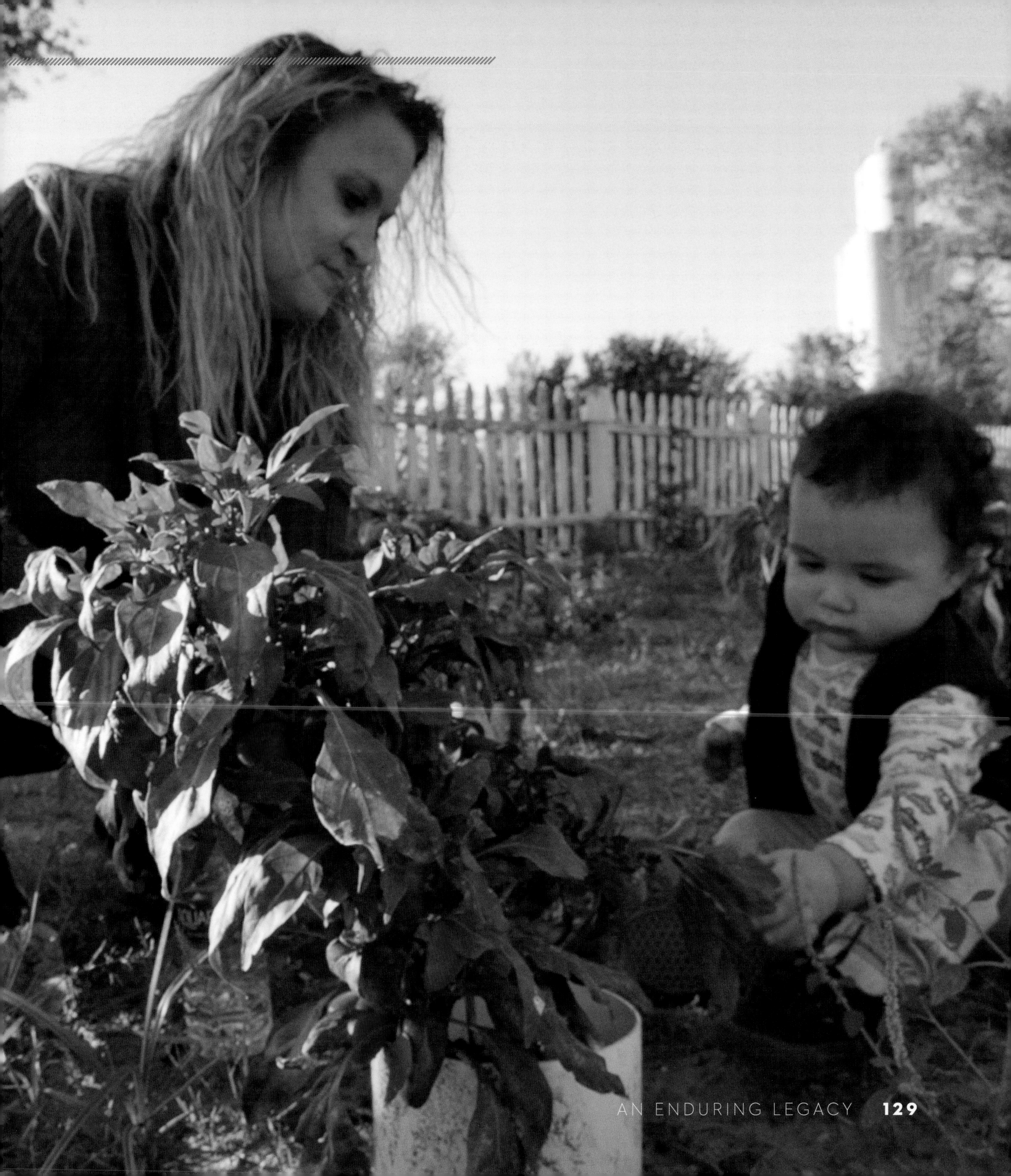

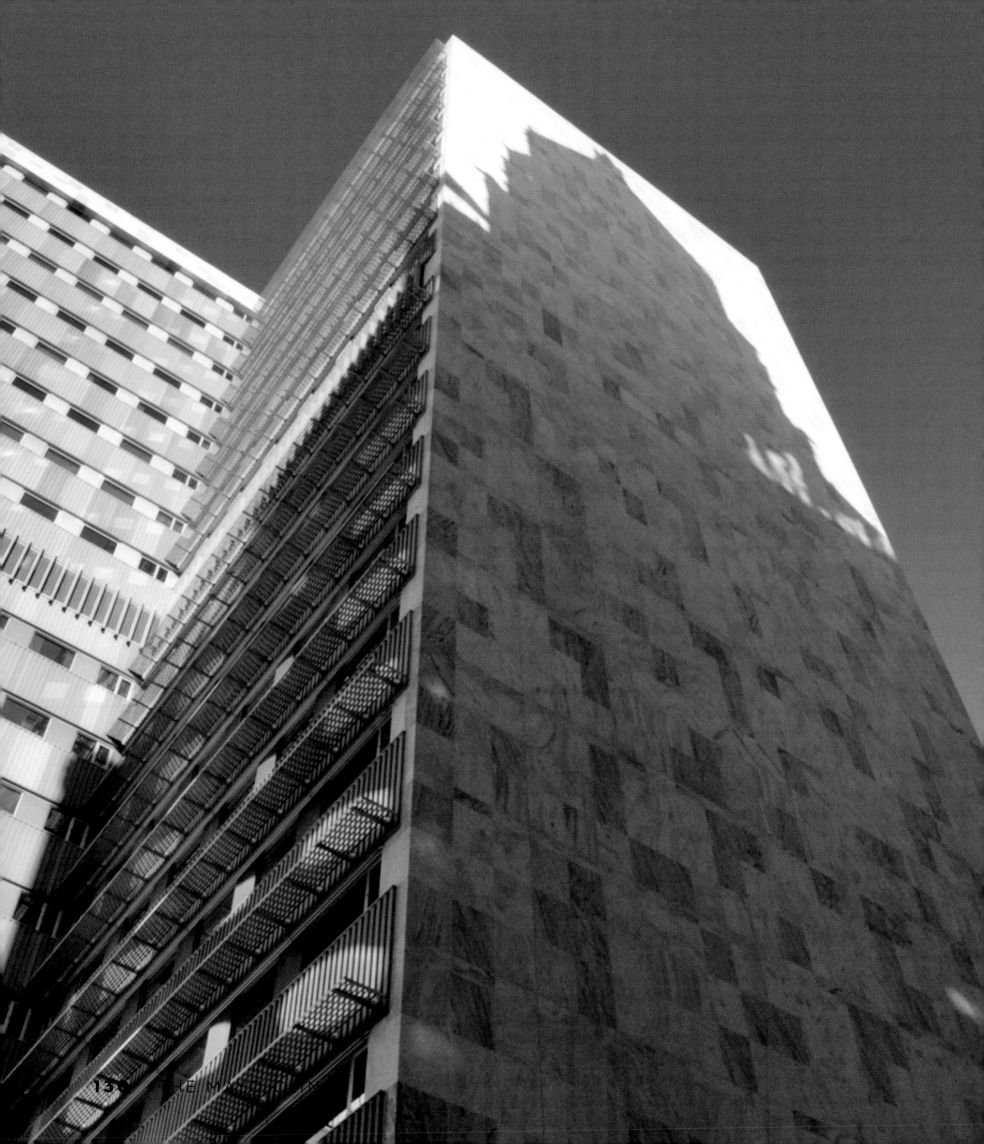

MAYO CLINIC TODAY AND TOMORROW

"Left open for further thought
and research."

"Patients are waiting."

More than 150 years separate these two statements, yet they express a shared commitment to serve humanity by continuously advancing medical science through research and education.

The first statement comes from William Worrall Mayo, M.D., in his handwritten notes, dating to 1866—the oldest medical records in Mayo Clinic's database, which now exceeds 10 million patient records. The second statement comes from Kendall Lee, M.D., Ph.D. A Mayo Clinic neurosurgeon, Dr. Lee describes how he and many colleagues use the statement to answer the question, "Why do you do research?"

This theme of change and continuity resonates in the film, *The Mayo Clinic: Faith, Hope, Science*, by the Ken Burns and Ewers Brothers production teams. W.W. Mayo's eldest son, William J. Mayo, M.D., wrote: "We have never been allowed to lose sight of the fact that the main purpose to be served by the Clinic is the care of the sick." The means by which Mayo Clinic provides care, however, continue to evolve and expand.

Mayo Clinic today is vastly different from the original consulting offices of Dr. W.W. Mayo and his sons, working with the Sisters of Saint Francis at Saint Marys Hospital about one mile away. Mayo is an internationally recognized, comprehensive, not-for-profit academic medical center and specialty group practice that provides inpatient and outpatient care on three campuses (Rochester, Minnesota; Jacksonville, Florida; and Scottsdale and Phoenix, Arizona) and the Mayo Clinic Health System, a network of regional community providers in Minnesota, Iowa, and Wisconsin. And in far-flung communities across the United States and around the globe, non-owned, affiliate organizations collectively known as Mayo Clinic Care Network collaborate with Mayo to extend its expertise to their patients and enhance the delivery of locally provided care. Mayo Clinic College of Medicine and Science has five schools with tens of thousands of alumni who practice throughout the world. Mayo Medical Laboratories, Mayo Clinic Global Business Solutions, and Mayo Clinic Social Media Network connect Mayo's expertise with patients, caregivers, news media, and business collaborators.

What has not changed is the mission—placing the needs of the patient first. This is the focus of everything Mayo does and its motivation for the future.

Some may think it odd that Mayo groups all of its work under the word Clinic, but it's truly apt. The schools and laboratories, along with the research and education staff, all contribute to patient care. The Mayos conceived of a place where research brings solutions to patients and training at the highest level advances the medical profession. That's why many Mayo Clinic physicians conduct research and teach in addition to caring for patients. Each endeavor drives and supports the others. Behind the description of a Mayo Clinic staff member as a "medical expert," there is an extensive list of published contributions to medicine and a long line of former students and trainees, in addition to a depth of diagnostic experience.

Just as the Mayo brothers traveled throughout the world to improve their medical knowledge, Mayo's faculty, staff, and students are encouraged to be lifelong learners. Scientists can become physicians; clinicians can become researchers. The medical school has one of the most competitive enrollment standards in the United States. Students are pushed to see the humanity—the patient perspective—in everything.

Robert Waller, M.D., emeritus president and CEO of Mayo Clinic, summed up this philosophy in six words: "Patients first, everyone matters, unconditional kindness." The philosophy is expressed in a variety of ways, all of which contribute to a unique environment of healing. The Mayo Clinic Model of Care includes the commitment that Mayo Clinic will provide an "unhurried examination of each patient." Dress and decorum standards allow expression of individuality for staff members within the context of professionalism and demonstration of respect for patients. Art, architecture, landscaping, and programs in the humanities are not "extras." They are embedded into the three-fold mission of patient care, research, and education.

In addition to its medical school, Mayo Clinic College of Medicine and Science includes Mayo Clinic Graduate School of Biomedical Sciences (research), Mayo Clinic School of Graduate Medical Education (residency program), Mayo Clinic School of Health Sciences (technical training), and Mayo Clinic School of Continuous Professional Development. All use unique approaches to education and are actively changing the way medicine is taught. There are classrooms, lecture halls, and labs. But, really, students, residents and fellows are everywhere, as are the staff physicians and scientists who also serve as faculty. One doesn't attend school at Mayo Clinic; one becomes part of Mayo Clinic. It follows that Mayo hires many of its own graduates.

Just as Will and Charlie Mayo learned from their father, some Mayo researchers can trace their lineage of training back three or four generations at the organization. Today, scientists and students learn from and build on the foundational discoveries of their mentors. More than a thousand physicians and medical scientists publish 7,000-plus articles, books, and other publications in the professional literature every year.

Mayo researchers are passionate about their work. Every day they pass patients on the sidewalks and in the hallways as they head to their labs. There is no better reminder of why they continue to discover, develop, and apply findings to answer the unmet needs of millions. In doing so, they change the practice of medicine, with new therapies and innovations.

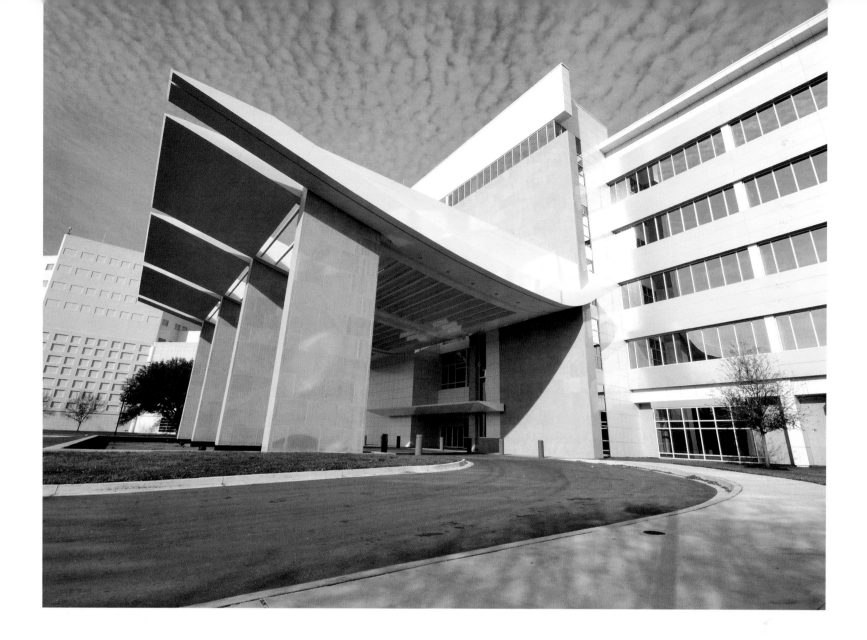

Mayo Clinic, which introduced CT scanning to North America, continues to advance medical imaging. International manufacturers send collaborators to work with Mayo radiology and ultrasound researchers. One outcome is magnetic resonance elastography, or MRE, which measures the stiffness of an organ inside the body. Another example is a simple, effective home screening test for colorectal cancer. Mayo is a leader in the new field of virus-based cancer therapies, which have been used successfully on ovarian, brain, and blood cancers. Mayo research in visualizing the brain has changed how researchers study Alzheimer's disease. One physician-researcher teamed up with a Mayo physicist to develop molecular breast imaging, a highly accurate tool that helps diagnose cancer in women with dense breast tissue.

Science happens in collaboration, not isolation. Mayo researchers work in teams that may include scientists from multiple disciplines, physicians engaged in research, medical residents and research fellows, graduate students, visiting scientists, technologists, technicians, bioinformatics experts, engineers, and a range of lab specialists. Mayo also collaborates with researchers from hundreds of other institutions around the world.

From discovery science—the basic cellular and molecular investigations in the laboratory—to animal and computer modeling and more than 12,000 active human studies, Mayo conducts medical science along the full range of discovery. Biomedical engineering and population studies play key roles, as does a field that Mayo effectively launched: the Science of Health Care Delivery. Henry Plummer, M.D., began studying and applying industrial engineering methods to the practice of medicine in the early twentieth century; he aligned its benefits to patient scheduling and the design of exam rooms and patient areas. Dr. Plummer's integration of medicine and engineering has grown into a joint research and clinical center that analyzes how Mayo practices medicine, and then implements improvements and efficiencies, all with the patient in mind. This is why, in many cases, a patient can arrive at Mayo Clinic for tests, have a diagnosis by the end of the day, and receive treatment the next morning.

Mayo Clinic is nationally ranked first in more medical disciplines than any other hospital. That speaks to depth of expertise in many areas, though it's the integration of specialties and the culture of collaboration that makes it possible to

Above: Florida campus
Opposite: Arizona campus

help patients with complex conditions. Physician specialists consulting in hallways, via electronic media, and over phone calls ensure that therapies don't conflict and that the person is getting the best overall care.

Just a few areas that are recognized for research expertise and quality of care are: endocrinology, diabetes and nutrition, rheumatology, infectious diseases, pediatrics, orthopedics, geriatrics, pulmonary and critical care, sports medicine, emergency medicine, gynecology, nephrology, urology, rehabilitation, psychiatry, gastroenterology, and ear-nose-throat specialties. Mayo's leadership in transplanting multiple organs at one time, the separation of conjoined twins, and its first full-face transplant are emblematic of multiple teams working together to plan, prepare, and resolve complex cases.

Mayo has long been a leader in neurology and neurosciences, whether in Alzheimer's and other dementias, epilepsy, multiple sclerosis, or Parkinson's and other tremor-related diseases. Researchers have discovered conditions that mask themselves as other illnesses and are often misdiagnosed, often developing tests to tell the difference. Cardiology and heart disease is a major field of expertise from diagnosis, repair, and transplant to development of heart valves, devices, and new medications. Mayo is known as a leader in cardiac clinical trials, often coordinating multisite studies.

Individualized or precision medicine is a Mayo strength in which knowledge of a person's genome is used to diagnose, predict, prevent, and treat a condition. Medical genomics began as research and has evolved into medical practice. Today the discipline uses genetic screening data to determine the cause of confusing symptoms or hard-to-diagnose diseases. Mayo pioneered the field of pharmacogenomics—using the right drug in the right dose at the right time, tailored to the individual patient. About 30 years ago, a Mayo researcher developed the first gene-based test to differentiate the subset of children with leukemia for whom the standard treatment had no effect. Today, that same approach is being used in many areas at Mayo. It is part of ongoing research and patient care, and will have a key role in the future of medicine.

Similarly, regenerative medicine, the science of encouraging organs to repair, regrow, or restore themselves, is another priority at Mayo Clinic. Laboratory studies and clinical trials are ongoing in more than 30 conditions. What's the best way to use a person's stem cells as a safe, effective prompt for other cells to repair or replace areas too damaged to function? That's the focus. Regenerative medicine goes beyond treating symptoms or the impairment left by a disease to helping the body heal itself. In the case of the heart, it means bringing the heart back to complete use following a heart attack; to make the damage disappear—to fully cure. Mayo already has regenerative medicine suites next to its surgical suites in one hospital and will be adding them to others.

These are only a handful of hundreds of areas where Mayo is making discoveries and translating them into patient care as quickly as it is safe to do so. Mayo is also collaborating with business more than ever before, through direct associations, joint research projects, consulting, or cooperatively commercializing the outcomes of Mayo's research discoveries. Mayo scientists are launching startup companies based on their research. Many of those firms can be found near Mayo Clinic campuses and elsewhere in the world.

At all campuses, Mayo has invested in growing its operations; in Minnesota, it has spurred expansion in Rochester with the Destination Medical Center initiative, a public-private economic development consortium and the largest in Minnesota's history. Nationally and internationally, partnerships with other centers are leading to new collaborations and advances. The most recent agreement is a partnership for medical practice, research, and education with the University of Oxford in the United Kingdom, formalized shortly before the two-hundredth anniversary of William Worrall Mayo's birth in Salford, England.

"People sometimes try to imagine what W.W. Mayo and his sons, and the first Franciscan Sisters, would say if they saw us now," says John Noseworthy, M.D., president and CEO of Mayo Clinic. "I think they'd be impressed by what twenty-first-century health care can do in service to humanity. I trust they'd be inspired by how much we look to their values and example in changing times. It would be a great conversation—and I'm sure they would ask, 'What are you doing next?'"

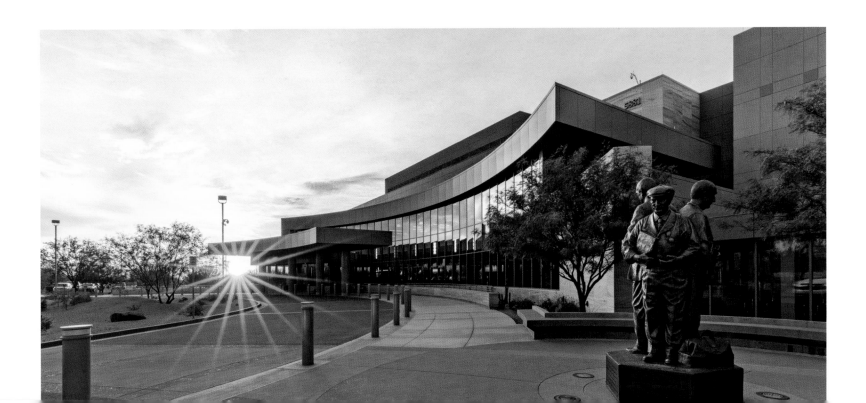

MAYO CLINIC TIMELINE

1819

William Worrall (W.W.) Mayo was born in England. He grew up with a love of science and a social conviction of giving back to others. He immigrated to the United States in 1846, earned two medical degrees, and married Louise Wright.

1828

Maria Moes was born in Luxembourg. She immigrated to the United States in 1851 and entered religious life. As Mother Alfred Moes, she founded two Franciscan congregations, one of which was located in Rochester, Minnesota.

1864

W.W. Mayo, M.D., opened a medical practice in Rochester. His sons, William James (Will) and Charles Horace (Charlie), graduated from medical school in the 1880s.

1883

A tornado devastated Rochester. The Franciscan Sisters and the Mayos cared for the wounded survivors. Afterward, Mother Alfred said the Sisters would build and staff a hospital if the Mayos provided medical care. Their agreement established a values-based collaboration that continues today.

1889

Saint Marys Hospital opened, using new antiseptic methods that made surgery much safer.

LATE 1800s–EARLY 1900s

The Mayos and their associates created a new model of medical care. They blended engineering principles with a humanistic ethos that placed the needs of the patient first in a culture of multispecialty teamwork.

1905

Louis Wilson, M.D., developed a method to freeze tissue specimens. This revolutionized surgery by making it possible to diagnose and remove tumors in one operation.

1906

Visiting physicians established the Surgeons Club, forerunner of Mayo Clinic College of Medicine and Science.

1907

Henry Plummer, M.D., created the unified medical record. Maud Mellish joined the Mayo practice, setting editorial standards that made Mayo a leader in medical publications. In 1926, she began the acclaimed medical journal, *Mayo Clinic Proceedings*. John Kahler, a local entrepreneur, founded a hospital that became Rochester Methodist Hospital in 1954.

1908

Harry Harwick joined the Mayo practice. He and Dr. Will Mayo created the model of physician-administrator collaboration that is a hallmark of Mayo Clinic today.

1914

Mayo Clinic opened the world's first building designed for multispecialty group practice. Its blend of efficiency and aesthetics set the standard for subsequent Mayo facilities.

1920

Albert Broders, M.D., developed an index to "grade" tumors by severity, which was adopted around the world.

1922

Russell Wilder, M.D., and colleagues conducted early clinical trials on insulin.

1934

President Franklin D. Roosevelt honored the Mayo brothers as "teachers of America."

1935

John Lundy, M.D., established the first blood bank in the United States.

1939

Both Mayo brothers and Sister Joseph Dempsey, longtime superintendent of Saint Marys Hospital, died within a few months of each other. Thanks to careful planning, the institution continued to thrive.

1941–1945

Mayo's World War II contributions included two Army hospital units in the South Pacific. Pioneering aero-medical research led to the G-Suit, high-altitude oxygen mask, and other innovations.

1942

Wallace Herrell, M.D., and colleagues published the first report in the United States medical literature on the systemic use of penicillin.

1945

William Feldman, D.V.M., and Corwin Hinshaw, Ph.D., M.D., conducted studies and clinical trials on streptomycin, proving the first successful drug therapy for tuberculosis.

1950

Edward Kendall, Ph.D., and Philip Hench, M.D., shared the Nobel Prize in Physiology or Medicine for the discovery of cortisone.

1955

John Kirklin, M.D., and colleagues helped pioneer open-heart surgery with the heart-lung bypass machine. Advances in heart surgery and innovations such as the post-anesthesia recovery room led to Mayo's early contributions in developing the intensive care unit.

1957

Mayo Clinic received its first research grant from the National Institutes of Health.

1969

Mark Coventry, M.D., performed the first hip implant with an FDA-approved artificial joint.

1973

Hillier Baker, M.D., brought the first CT scanner in North America to Mayo Clinic.

National Cancer Institute designated Mayo Clinic as an NCI Cancer Center.

1980s

Mayo Clinic began diversification initiatives that included publishing consumer-based health information (1983); integrating with Saint Marys Hospital and Rochester Methodist Hospital (1986); opening in Jacksonville, Florida (1986); opening in Scottsdale (1987) and Phoenix (1998), Arizona; establishing Mayo Clinic Health System in the Upper Midwest (1992); and establishing Mayo Clinic Care Network (2011).

2001

Mayo developed a one-hour test to detect anthrax poisoning.

2003

Mayo was recognized as the nation's first Comprehensive Cancer Center with sites in Arizona, Florida, and Minnesota.

2004

Mayo Clinic researchers were the first to model the SARS virus.

2011

Mayo established transformational centers in individualized and regenerative medicine and the science of health-care delivery.

2016

Proton beam cancer therapy centers opened in Minnesota and Arizona.

Surgeons successfully conducted Mayo's first full face transplant; Mayo chosen to host the national "All of Us" biobank by National Institutes of Health.

2017

Mayo welcomed its first medical school class in Arizona.

2018

Integration of Mayo's current and historic medical records into a single, organization-wide, comprehensive electronic medical record system.

FILM CREDITS

DIRECTED BY
KEN BURNS
ERIK EWERS
CHRISTOPHER LOREN
EWERS

WRITTEN BY
DAVID BLISTEIN
KEN BURNS

PRODUCED BY
JULIE COFFMAN

CO-PRODUCED BY
ERIK EWERS
CHRISTOPHER LOREN
EWERS

EDITED BY
ERIK EWERS A.C.E.

**DIRECTOR OF
PHOTOGRAPHY**
CHRISTOPHER LOREN
EWERS

ORIGINAL MUSIC BY
DAVID CIERI

NARRATED BY
PETER COYOTE

VOICES
TOM HANKS
Will Mayo
SAM WATERSTON
Charlie Mayo
KEVIN CONWAY
William Worrall Mayo

OTHER VOICES
BLYTHE DANNER
GENE JONES
CAROLYN McCORMICK
JOSH LUCAS
ROSA GILMORE

**SENIOR HISTORICAL
CONSULTANT**
W. BRUCE FYE, M.D.

ASSISTANT PRODUCERS
ALI SCATTERGOOD
SAMANTHA SPIELBERG

ASSISTANT EDITOR
ALI SCATTERGOOD

**POST-PRODUCTION
ASSISTANT**
REBECCA CONNOLLY

FIELD PRODUCER
MARIAH A. DORAN

TECHNICAL DIRECTOR
DAVE MAST

**POST-PRODUCTION
SUPERVISOR**
DANIEL J. WHITE

**CHIEF FINANCIAL
OFFICER**
JENNIFER FABIS

**ACCOUNTANT
FOR KEN BURNS**
CHRISTOPHER SINK

**COORDINATING
PRODUCER FOR
KEN BURNS**
ELLE CARRIÈRE

**ASSISTANT
COORDINATING
PRODUCER FOR
KEN BURNS**
JILLIAN HEMPSTEAD

**ASSISTANTS
TO KEN BURNS**
CHRISTOPHER DARLING
CAULEY POWELL

**THE BETTER
ANGELS SOCIETY**
AMY MARGERUM BERG,
President
COURTNEY CHAPIN,
Executive Director

**ADDITIONAL
CINEMATOGRAPHY**
ALEX HADJILOUKAS
ALLEN MOORE

ASSISTANT CAMERA
ALEX HADJILOUKAS
PETER CATY
INÉS PORTUGAL

DRONE FOOTAGE
ADAM PASS
PETER CATY
PETE PALLAGI
RON PORTER
MICHAEL WHITTIER
JEFF PRESTON
CLIF BREWER

SOUND RECORDING
SERGIO REYES-
SHEEHAN
RICHARD BUONAGURIO
ALEX HADJILOUKAS

**SUPERVISING
SOUND EDITOR**
ERIK EWERS

SOUND EDITORS
ERIK EWERS
DAVE MAST
RYAN GIFFORD
BRYAN PUGH

**SOUND POST-
PRODUCTION**
SOUNDTRACK NEW
YORK, NY

RE-RECORDING MIXER
DOMINICK TAVELLA
CHRIS CHAE

**VOICE-OVER
RECORDING**
LOU VERRICO
DAVE WEISSMAN
CITYVOX, NEW YORK,
NY
GRAHAM STONE
STONE STUDIOS, CT

**DIGITAL IMAGE
RESTORATION**
EVAN BARLOW

**DIGITAL ANIMATION &
GRAPHIC EFFECTS**
BRIAN LEE

GRAPHICS AND TITLING
JULIE COFFMAN

**INTERMEDIATE SERVICES
PROVIDED BY**
TECHNICOLOR
POSTWORKS NY

DI COLORIST
JACK LEWARS

DI CONFORM EDITOR
JEFF CORNELL

**ADDITIONAL CONFORM
EDITORS**
RYAN MCMAHON
SEAN PERRY

DI PRODUCER
KYLE CASEY

FILM SCANNING
JAKE CAFFERA

DIGITAL RESTORATION
BRIAN WOOS
ROSS HENDRICKSON

**CHIEF TECHNOLOGY
OFFICER**
JOE BEIRNE

CHIEF SALES OFFICER
CAROL JAZWINSKI

**VP OF CREATIVE
SERVICES**
BENJAMIN MURRAY

**TRANSCRIPTION
SERVICES**
SARA HALEY
JULIE HONEA

CATERING SERVICES
SUSAN ROGERS
SUSAN DUPREY
JOAN BALLA

PRODUCTION INTERNS
REBECCA CONNOLLY
SPENCER WALD

LEGAL SERVICES
DREW PATRICK
MICHAEL McCORMACK
MAAYAN ZACH
JEREMY S. GOLDMAN

MUSICIAN
DAVID CIERI, *piano*

ADDITIONAL MUSICIANS
DANIEL BRANTIGAN,
flugelhorn
JAY FREDERICK,
percussion
MIKE BROWN, *bass*
PUTNAM MURDOCK,
guitar
RUBIN KODHELI, *cello*
YOKO WAYNEN, *violin*
BILL FRISELL, *guitar*

MUSIC PRODUCED BY
ERIK EWERS

MUSIC RECORDED AT
FIGURE 8 RECORDING,
Brooklyn, NY

MUSIC ENGINEER
BRYAN PUGH

ADDITIONAL MUSIC
"Battle Cry of Freedom"
Composer: George
Frederick Root
Performed by Jacqueline
Schwab

"The Ragtime Dance"
Composer: Scott Joplin
Performed by Jacqueline
Schwab

"Partita in D minor for
solo violin"
Composer: Johann
Sebastian Bach
Performed by Roger Frisch

"Appalachian Spring"
Written by Aaron Copland
Published by Boosey &
Hawkes, sole licensee
Courtesy of the Aaron
Copland Fund for
Music, Inc.
Performed by The
Czechoslovak Radio
Symphony
Orchestra, Courtesy of
Naxos of America, Inc.

"Hard Times"
Composer: Stephen Foster
Performed by Jacqueline
Schwab

"A Psalm of Life"
Written by Charles
Beecher
Performed by Martin
Simpson-Guitar and Joe
Weed-Fiddle Courtesy
of Gourd Music (BMI) /
Jozone Music (BMI)

ARCHIVAL FOOTAGE
Division of Media Support
Services, Mayo Clinic,
Rochester, MN
National Archives and
Records Administration

**ARCHIVAL
PHOTOGRAPHS**
Michelle Andrews, Kaiser
Health News
AP Images
AP Photo/Harvey Georges
Assisi Heights Archives,
Sisters of Saint Francis,
Rochester, Minnesota
Melinda Beck, The Wall
Street Journal
Henry P. Bosse
Beth and Scott Brasseur
Cajal Institute, Spanish
National Research
Council, (CSIC)
Madrid, Spain
Christy Ford Chapin, Tim
Lahan, The New York
Times
Connecticut Historical
Society
Dartmouth Library
Special Collections
Alyssa and Christopher
Feenstra
Roger Frisch
W. Bruce Fye, M.D.
W. Bruce Fye Center for
the History of Medicine,
Rochester, MN
Getty Images
Harvard Medical Library
in the Francis A.
Countway Library of
Medicine
The History Center of
Olmsted County
Howard Lipin/U-T San
Diego/Zuma Press, The
Wall Street Journal
Anna Jenkins
Lyndon B. Johnson
Presidential Library and
Museum
Shannon Leon
Library of Congress,
Prints and Photographs
Division

The Lillian and Clarence
de la Chapelle Medical
Archives at NYU
Los Angeles Times
Gail Manning and David
Richards
Mayo Architectural and
Engineering Design
Services
The Minnesota Historical
Society
The Minnesota Historical
Society Newspaper Hub
National Archives and
Records Administration
The New York Public
Library, Astor, Lenox
and Tilden Foundations
Northwest Architectural
Archive
OHSU Historical
Collections & Archives
Otis Historical Archives,
National Museum of
Health and Medicine
Photographs © Stanley B.
Burns, MD & The Burns
Archive
Saint Marys Hospital
Archives, Rochester,
MN
Karl Schenk
Kelvin Smith University
Archives, Special
Collections
University of Michigan
Bentley Historical
Library
University of Minnesota
Archives, University of
Minnesota—Twin Cities
US National Library of
Medicine
Wellcome Images
Collection

**THE FILMMAKERS
WISH TO THANK**
Patricia Barrier, M.D.
Christopher Boes, M.D.
Sarah Botstein
Robert Brown, M.D.
L.A. Burdick's, Walpole,
NH, Sara Hatfield
Sarah Burns & David
McMahon
Lilly, Olivia & Willa Burns
Emily Christopherson
Dan, Casie and Clayton
Coffman
Matthew Dacy
Amy Davis
Dayton Duncan
Julie Dunfey
Christy, Billie and
Finnegan Ewers
Susan, Allie and Haley
Ewers
Gianrico Farrugia, M.D.
Virginia Fidel

Mark Flaherty
Florentine Films Editing
House
Florentine Films Brooklyn
Office
Jason Fortin
Paul, Lindsay, Adam and
AJ Frucci
Chris Gade
Kathryn Gatliff
Katy Haas
Sandra J. Hanson
Adeline Hofer
The Inn at Valley Farms,
Walpole, NH
Krista Lewis
Mayo Clinic Historic
Properties
Mayo Clinic Jacksonville,
FL
Mayo Clinic Public Affairs
Mayo Clinic Rochester,
MN
Mayo Clinic Scottsdale,
AZ
Peter Miller
John Murphy
Robert Nellis
John Noseworthy, M.D.
Lynn Novick
Wendy O'Connell
Karl Oestreich
Kerry Olsen, M.D.
The People of Walpole,
New Hampshire
Ginger Plumbo
Charles Potter
Megan Ruffe
Emily Schneider
Gary Sieck, Ph.D.
Sisters of St. Francis,
Rochester, MN
Susanna Steisel
Gary Stiller
Pam Tubridy Baucom
Bill and Chris Tugeau
Jonah Velasco
John T. Wald, M.D.
David Weiss
Sister Ellen Whelan,
O.S.F.
Renee Ziemer

SPECIAL THANKS
Allen Aksamit Jr., M.D.
Trish Amundson
Steven Arcieri
Niels Arnesen
Nicole Babcock
Dave Bartell
Bradey Bearden
LaVonne C. Beck
Atta Behfar, M.D., Ph.D.
Thomas S. Behrens
Kevin Bennet
Jo Bernal
Shantice Berry, RN
Emily Blahnik
Erwin Borgen
Soulmaz Boroumand, Ph.D.

Judy Boughey, M.D.
Fran Bowen
Matthew Brody
Tom Brokaw
Kenneth Brown
Alicen Buck
John Butz
Tina Byers
Tony Carlson
Jennifer Carroll
Mary Casalino
Vicki Chambard Torkelson
Chester's
Jered Chinnock
Gina M. Chiri-Osmond
Susannah Ciernia
Tony Cloer
Gerardo Colon-Otero,
M.D.
Dave Curtis
Joseph Dearani, M.D.
Quiana DeBrill, L.P.N.
Vickie Delaney
Allison Diamond
Doubletree by Hilton,
Rochester, MN
John Downer
Dina I. Drubach
Geraldine Farrugia
Alyssa Feenstra
Christopher Feenstra
Roger Frisch
Sr. Generose Gervais
GO Rochester Direct
Peter J. Grahn, Ph.D.
Eddie Greene, M.D.
Ethan Grove
Ernie Hain
Judith Hartzell
Hilton Garden Inn,
Rochester, MN
Erik Hyman
Anna, David, Marti &
Quinn Jenkins
Pamela Johnson, RN
Jacque Jones
Randall S. Jones
April Josselyn
Jay Kane
Molly Karus, RN
Jean Keane
Charlene Kelly
Fran & Marion Kelly
Kathleen Kennelly, M.D.,
Ph.D.
Sameer Keole, M.D.
Jean Klavetter
Jeanne Klein
Kim Klein
Michelle Klemm
Ramona Klemm
Brandon Knowles
John Kruesel
Dennis Lagerlof
Dalai Lama
Krystal Lamb
Igor A. Lavrov
Heather Lawton
Kendall Lee, M.D., Ph.D.
Shannon Leon

Glenn Lyden—PA
Rhoda Madson
Gail Manning
Samir Mardini, M.D.
Charles Mayo, II
John McCain
James McVeigh
Gary Meyerhofer
Minneapolis Orchestra:
Gwen Pappas
Emma Plehal
Stanislaw
Skrowaczewski
Siddhartha Mukherjee,
M.D., Ph.D.
Sr. Antoine Murphy
Carole Adrienne Murphy
Bradly Narr, M.D.
Heidi Nelson, M.D.
Jessica Nelson
Timothy Niewold, M.D.
Pat Noseworthy
Julian Ortiz
Larry Patnode
Bonnie Potter
Michael Potts
Jose Pulido, M.D.
Production Junction:
Chris Edwards
Mariah Honecker
Andy Marva
Dave McGrath
Theresa Sagan
Kevin Punsky
Dale Reed
Andrew Rhodes
Deborah Rhodes, M.D.
David Richards
Kate Richards
Louise Richards
Edward Rosenow III, M.D.
Jillian Roseone
Shawn Ruechel
Andrew Saunders
Nancy and Karl Schenk
Matthew C. Senjem
Zach Serres
Mike Shappell
Rafael Sierra, M.D.
Craig A. Smoldt
Rory Smoot, M.D.
Marta Solano, RN
Tiffany Staudacher
Robyn Stecher
Anne Steele
Terrie M. Stephans
Rosemary Stevens
Shannon Szecsy
Tenzin Taklha
James Taylor
Terry and Jean Taylor
Tessa's Office
Andre Terzic, M.D., Ph.D.
Sharon Theimer
Jason Tlusty
Andrew Tofilon
Gail Tostenson
Tricia Treuter
Mari Charisse Trinidad,
M.D.

Sr. Tierney Trueman
Mark Truty, M.D.
Jonah Velasco
Dean Von Bank
Michelle Wald
Courtney Walton
Sr. Lauren Weinandt
Lilli Mayo Weivoda
Kate Welp, RN
Sr. Ellen Whelan
Michael Whittier
Jordan Young
Katelyn Young
Peter Zimmerman

NATIONAL PUBLICITY
DKC PUBLIC RELATIONS
JOE DePLASCO & BRIAN
MORIARTY

**PRODUCED IN
ASSOCIATION WITH**
WETA WASHINGTON, DC

**EXECUTIVE IN CHARGE
OF PRODUCTION
FOR WETA**
DALTON DELAN

**PROJECT EXECUTIVE
FOR WETA**
ANNE HARRINGTON

PRODUCER FOR WETA
JIM CORBLEY

**FOUNDATION
DEVELOPMENT
FOR WETA**
ELAINE LAUGHLIN

**PRESIDENT & CEO
OF WETA**
SHARON ROCKEFELLER

A Production of Florentine
Films & Ewers Brothers
Productions

EXECUTIVE PRODUCER
KEN BURNS

© 2018 The Mayo Clinic
Film Project, LLC

FUNDING FOR THE FILM

Funding for *The Mayo Clinic* was provided by the following members of The Better Angels Society, a nonprofit organization dedicated to educating Americans about their history through documentary film:

Jay Alix & Una Jackman, Stephen and Barbara Slaggie and Family, The Russell and Carla Paonessa Family, Sandra and Bert Getz, GHR Foundation, The Pfeil Foundation, and Gilchrist and Amy Berg. Additional funding was provided by The Arthur Vining Davis Foundations.

ACKNOWLEDGMENTS

The authors are indebted to the highly professional multispecialty team that brought this book to life:

At Time Inc. Books, Sarah Rutledge adapted the script and oversaw the editorial process from start to finish; Jon Chaiet created a beautiful design that complemented the film and gave it a new dimension; April Colburn kept everyone on track with the schedule; and Nina Reed kept the partners on the same page.

At Ewers Brothers Productions, Rebecca Connolly responded to countless requests for information, images, and feedback.

At Mayo Clinic, Christopher Frye coordinated all the constantly moving pieces and kept the project moving; Matthew Dacy and Robert Nellis ensured accuracy; Erika Riggin worked tirelessly to confirm photo rights; and Chris Gade ensured timely access to Mayo resources.

Last but certainly not least, special thanks to our publisher, Arthur Klebanoff at RosettaBooks, for making this book possible.

INDEX

PHOTOGRAPHY CREDITS

Front cover: Christopher Loren Ewers

Back cover: Used with permission of Mayo Foundation for Medical Education and Research, all rights reserved

4-5, 14 top, 15 bottom, 16, 18 bottom, 20, 22, 26, 37 top left, 37 top right, 49 top, 50 left, 51 left, 53 left, 54 top, 55 top, 60, 62 top left, 62 top right, 62 bottom right, 63, 64 top, 65, 66 top, 67, 68 top, 69 bottom, 70, 74, 76 top, 77, 78, 79 top, 80, 81 top left, 81 bottom, 82, 83 top, 84, 88, 90 top, 90 bottom, 91 right, 92, 93 top, 94, 95 top, 95 center, 95 bottom, 96 top, 96 bottom left, 97, 99, 102, 104 top, 104 bottom, 105, 106, 108, 109 top left, 109 center right, 109 bottom, 111, 112, 118 left, 118 center, 118 right, 119 second from top, 119 second from bottom, 119 bottom, 120 top, 121, 122 bottom, 125 top left: used with permission of Mayo Foundation for Medical Education and Research, all rights reserved

2: Library of Congress

6, 14 bottom, 15 top, 17, 18 top, 19 bottom, 21, 23, 24-25 top, 24 bottom, 25 bottom, 40, 41, 42, 43 top, 43 bottom, 44 top, 44 bottom, 57, 58 top, 58 second from top, 58 second from bottom, 58 bottom, 59 top, 59 bottom, 69 top, 71, 72 top, 72 second from top, 72 second from bottom, 72 bottom, 73, 69 top, 71, 72 top, 72 second from top, 72 second from bottom, 72 bottom, 73, 83 bottom, 85, 86 top, 86 center, 86 bottom, 87 top, 87 bottom, 98, 100, 101 top, 101 center left, 101 center right, 101 bottom left, 101 bottom right, 107 top, 107 bottom, 110, 113, 114 top, 114 center, 114 bottom, 115 top, 115 second from top, 115 second from bottom, 115 bottom, 116, 124 top, 124 bottom, 125 top right, 125 bottom, 126, 127, 128 bottom, 129, 130: Christopher Loren Ewers

9: Malgorzata Weivoda

10: Jodi Olson

13: Evan W. Barlow

19 top: The Bettman Collection/Getty Images

28: The Detroit Publishing Company Photograph Collection, Library of Congress

29: Russell Lee, Farm Security Administration—Office of War Information Photograph Collection, Library of Congress

30 top: Disabled American Veterans of the World War, Prints and Photographs Division, Library of Congress

30 bottom, 31 top: Wellcome Images Collection

31 bottom: Herbert Merton Greene Papers, Historical Images Collection, Historical Images Collection, OHSU Historical Collections & Archives

32, 38 top, 54 bottom: The Minnesota Historical Society

33: Beth and Scott Brasseur

34, 35: James F. Gibson, The Civil War Collection, Library of Congress

36 top: The Civil War Collection, Library of Congress

36 bottom: ©Stanley B. Burns, MD & The Burns Archive

37 bottom: The Bettman Collection/Getty Images

38 bottom: FotoSoyuz/Hulton Archive/Getty Images

39 left: Byron Collection/Museum of the City of New York/Getty Images

39 right: U.S. National Library of Medicine

45: Alyssa and Christopher Feenstra

46, 48, 49 center, 49 bottom, 50 right, 55 bottom, 62 bottom left, 68 bottom: The History Center of Olmsted County

51 right: Ullstein Bild collection/Getty Images

52 top: University of Michigan Bentley Historical Library

52 bottom: Charles Milton Bell, Library of Congress

53 right: Herbert A. French, National Photo Company, Library of Congress

56: Yael Joel/The Life Picture Collection/Getty Images

64 bottom: Assisi Heights Archives, Sisters of Saint Francis, Rochester, Minnesota

66 bottom: Kirn Vintage Stock/Corbis Historical Collection/Getty Images

76 bottom: Mutahara Mobashar, Library of Congress

79 bottom: Harvard Medical Library in the Francis A. Countway Library of Medicine

81 top right: Library of Congress

91 left: Ewers Brothers Productions, llc

93 bottom: Wright Brothers Negatives, Library of Congress

96 bottom right: Courtesy of University of Minnesota Archives, University of Minnesota—Twin Cities

109 top right, 109 center left: Alfred Eisenstaedt, The Life Picture Collection, Getty Images

119 top: John Vachon, Farm Security Administration—Office of War Information Photograph Collection, Library of Congress

120 bottom: Gail Manning and David Richards (Claire); Lakewood Cemetery, Minneapolis, MN (gravestone)

122 top: Earl Theisen, Prints and Photographs Division, Library of Congress

123 top: The LBJ Presidential Library/Library of Congress

123 center: J. Scott Applewhite/Los Angeles Times

123 bottom: NurPhoto Collection/Getty Images

128 top: Shannon Leon personal photos

132: Dan Hubert

133: Pete Pallagi